Unfold Me

Jenn,

Remember there is always hope.

Love & Light

XO

Dee.

Unfold Me

DEIRDRE MALONEY

Dedication

Dedicated to my family:
Jon, your love, guidance, and vision have offered me
unwavering strength and support. You are the love of my life.

Monika, Charlize, Jonathan, and Kayden, I write this book
to set the example of true self-acceptance. No matter what
happens in life, you can always try one more time.

Contents

Part 1: Fear

Part 2: Shame

Part 3: Wholehearted

PART ONE

Fear

The first women's Healing Circle I attended in 2017 was the catalyst to my healing journey. The group was led into a meditative state and asked to imagine ourselves as young girls, tuning into our emotions as we walked through a forest. I was six years old, and it was a beautiful day. The sun shone through the leaves of the trees around me, and they glittered from the movement created by the breeze. I felt very sad and lonely. Nobody cared about me, and I felt unprotected and vulnerable. I looked up at the magnificent beauty surrounding me, and I felt so small. A profound question lingered in my mind; why didn't anyone love me? I sobbed as I left the guided meditation that had split my heart wide open. The time to revisit the beginning had arrived.

1

The Beginning

I was born in 1980 in rural New Brunswick in New Castle. My parents each had a son from a previous relationship, and both boys were eleven years older than myself. I also had a brother who was one year older than me, my parents' first child together. With the hope of creating a better life, my father left when I was a year old and went to Toronto to find work. Within six months, my father found decent employment, and my mother brought the three of us with her on the train to Toronto, leaving the home my father had built for us. Her son lived with us, and my dad's son lived in British Columbia with his mother. We didn't see him very often. My mother found work after we arrived in Toronto, and I was sent with my siblings to an in-home daycare. I was shuffled through a few daycares in my younger years, and I don't have any good memories from those experiences. We walked and took the bus when we were really small with my Mom hurrying us along so she could get to work.

On the rainy days, I remember being terrified of the worms that would swarm the sidewalks, forcing my mother to carry me because I held my ground and screamed relentlessly, terrified I would step on one if I moved. Eventually, she got a little wagon, and she pulled me around in it on those gloomy days to keep me safe from the wicked worms.

My mother's biological father died in a car accident after a night of drinking when Mom was ten, no money to his name except the $40 in his wallet. My grandmother was now a young widow and had four mouths to feed. With Mom being the oldest, she looked after all of her siblings while her mother went to work.

Extremely shy as a young girl, I always hid behind my mother, hoping it would render me invisible. I hid from everyone: even Grandpa, Mother's stepfather, though most kids would. He was loud and rude, and to this day, I believe he enjoyed scaring me. He was in the Navy and had thick skin and a quick tongue. Compassion and empathy lived beneath his boot and never saw the light of day. I always wondered what my grandmother had seen in him. She must have been in desperate need of help and companionship to take him in.

When I was young, my mother allowed me to use her as a shield, and I tucked myself safely behind her. Now, I suppose she was only extending her own protection. At the time, however, I didn't understand it in this way. In my eyes, my mom was a queen: beautiful, brave, desirable, and a brilliant hostess who held down the house, which was always in order, all while working a full-time job. She had dark, luscious brown hair, olive skin, slim legs that seemed to go on for miles, and deep brown eyes. Any time I hear the song "Brown-Eyed Girl" by Van Morrison, I think of how she must have been as a teenager when the song was released in the late sixties, free-spirited and wildly mystical. Of course, this was my imagination and probably far from reality, knowing she got pregnant with my oldest brother at seventeen. I saw the way men looked at her, including my grandfather. This became my first introduction to sex appeal.

As a child, I desperately wanted my mother's love and attention. I don't have many memories of tender moments shared with her. Whenever I came to her for a random affectionate hug or wanted to run my fingers through her hair, I was greeted with a flutter of hands pushing me away. Shooing me, not like you would a bee or spider, more like you would to a cobweb: quick, irritated, and with a hint of silly. The silly part, I believe, was added to soften the blow. She had no idea she was thickening the walls of my cocoon.

My dad adored me on occasion. I drank it up obviously. "Babykins" was what he called me—with a big smile and warm blue eyes. I called him "Daddy-too." Dad really wasn't around much, and when he was, he tended to be a bit of a lone wolf. He preferred puttering around in his workshop or reading the newspaper over games and books with the kids. He and my mother often fought about money and expenses. She couldn't abide by a budget and felt entitled to her shopping expenditures regardless of how much money they had in the bank. This was one terrible quality I would later bring into my own marriage. However, there were great attributes she passed along, like cooking, baking, and interior decorating. She was my first role model in leading a healthy lifestyle, exercising with me in the form of walks and Jane Fonda videotapes. Yes, we wore the pastel spandex gymnast outfits.

Dad was the soft one, leaving the discipline to my mother. She scolded, yelled, and was after us constantly, especially if she was cleaning. She paddled us the odd time as small children, though she mostly resorted to pinching, which, in public, gave her immediate control and prevented anyone noticing the interaction that left me scared, angry, and retreating further into myself.

I was a loner in school. We moved a lot. Mom always wanting bigger, better, more. Changing schools every one to two years and being forced to try fitting in all over again was something I was terrible at as a child. I absolutely dreaded going to school, feared recess and lunch, and often found refuge in the girls' bathroom until my lonely walk home to the kitchen for a Twinkie or grilled cheese sandwich. This was the start of a mild eating disorder that would follow me into my thirties. Drowning out the discomfort of the day with food was easy and satisfying. Stuff it in, satiate the senses, and numb the pain.

What a dark cycle it is to overeat in place of communication and connection. The feelings of self-loathing and disgust are strong once the stuffed belly begins to ache. Later on, I set a special day aside for my binge-eating and starved myself all week in anticipation of the big feed.

Alongside my obsession with food, I also had precocious puberty. This condition gave me the pubic hair and bone structure of a twelve-year-old at the age of six, which is what led my mother to look into it. I occasionally went to Sick Kids Hospital in Toronto for tests, pokes, and prods to see what they could do to slow down my growth. She feared I would grow so fast and then stop before I had reached five feet. Every night, I took an intramuscular shot of some concoction meant to slow my growth. The nightly injections lasted about a year before my mother couldn't bear to give one more as I cried and begged not to do them. We let nature take its course, and here I am at 5'3, the average height of a woman. The condition brought me a lot of attention. Of course, this also left me feeling fat. As a young girl, I held a thick figure, and I called myself fat, along with my brothers, but looking back, I don't see that I was at all. From grades four to six, I was a full foot taller than the other girls and had the breasts and hips of a sixteen-year-old next to flat and straight. Because I was the first to hit puberty, by nine years old I'd started my period.

I remember being in Florida for my tenth birthday. We were at a water park; god, I was excited to be there. Unfortunately, I got my period, and my mother tried to teach me how to insert a tampon from the opposite side of the bathroom door in the hotel room. She asked me to stick it in the hole between my legs. "It's easy," she said. "Get one foot up on the toilet seat and relax." I wondered what this hole looked like and where it was.

Nobody had ever spoken of this hole before. I tried to figure it out, but without a diagram, I didn't have a clue what I was looking for! "Mom, this is not happening! I just don't know what to do," I said, defeated.

"Just stay in the water; you won't bleed if you're in the water," she advised. Thank the high heavens it was true, at least on that day.

Back at school, the boys were very curious, and I got grabbed, poked, and prodded once again. I wasn't sure what to think of all the attention. Part of me was flattered, but another part didn't like to be set apart from the other girls. It was like I was a bit of a freak show out for others' entertainment, and it left an emptiness in my soul. Again, I didn't fit in. Would I ever?

At nine years old, my childhood ended when I was molested. It is a memory etched in my mind with perfect clarity and something that sent me on a downward spiral. He was a grown man, and I had never felt afraid or uncomfortable around him. He called me into a bedroom at home, and I came bumbling along, curious to see what he wanted.

He said, "Come on in—have a seat" and gestured toward the bed. The next thing I knew, he was on top of me.

I giggled at first, thinking he was horsing around, and I said, "You're going to squish me flat like a pancake." Suddenly, he started to feel very heavy. As soon as the words had left my mouth, panic struck through me like lightning, and my thoughts raced. *What is happening? Why is he dry-humping my leg? Holy shit, I can feel his erection. This is bad.* My next words were "no, please get off me." I struggled to breathe, both from his weight and the panic at what I couldn't stop from happening. *I'm just a little girl. How did I get myself into this situation?*

He seemed to snap out of it and rolled off, allowing me to get up. I scurried to the front of the bed, extremely embarrassed, head hung, and utterly unsure of what to do or where to look. I didn't rush out of the bedroom because I was already frightened of hurting someone's feelings. So, I sat still and waited for dismissal or, better yet, for him to leave the room. He came to sit next to me instead. *Shit.* His hand went to my lap and made its way between my legs and started rubbing what I now know to be my clitoris. Feelings arose that I had never felt before, something inside me was being woken, and I knew this was very bad. I wanted to leave my body and escape my skin. The fear of everything I'd ever known to be true was ripped away from me.

I heard him speak, and I froze with fear. He asked, "Does this feel good?" *How can he ask me this question?* I felt so small and weak but managed to summon the simple word *no*, and he stopped. It was over.

He got up and left the room. Relief, shame, and sadness rushed over me in unbearable waves. I don't remember what I did next, but I have a feeling it was the beginning of many long hours I would spend alone in my room, completely disconnected from my family. I subconsciously decided to turn my inner self off because I could not handle the pain.

This was the biggest betrayal of my life. I felt I had been tossed aside, an old sweater that didn't fit right anymore. I was now an outcast in the family, and I played the role well. This marked the end of my childhood and the beginning of a sinister new decade.

This dirty little secret was kept for two years. I tucked it away as deep as I could, swearing to myself I would never speak of it. The incident disgusted me and made me feel vile. I couldn't relive that kind of shame. I often wondered how my mom never noticed me go into darkness, withdrawn and sombre, forever hiding in my room. My love for books ignited during this time; I loved being swept away in a good novel, and I spent hours and days in my room drifting away to another life, to someone else's story.

I still managed to have a good social life at this time. We spent two years in this home, and I developed some strong friendships. I often had sleepovers at friends' houses and met up with them at the park or went for a bike ride. It was common for us to go skating on weekends at the local community centre. Winters in Canada are harsh, extremely cold, and full of snow and ice. Getting into winter sports is one of the only ways to survive it. My parents often took us skiing, which I loved, even after having a big crash into a tree on one occasion that left me with a badly sprained ankle.

Skiing was a family outing. My parents, brother, and I headed up together; our parents went off to do their thing, and my brother and I went off to do ours. Skating, on the other hand, was never a family event. Only in the beginning, while we were learning, did our parents come to the arena. After that, they dropped us off at the front entrance for an afternoon with friends, or so everyone's parents thought.

At the age of ten, I'd gone completely boy crazy, desperately seeking the attention and affection of the opposite sex. Being at the rec centre gave me lots of opportunities to seek out a possible boyfriend. There were always lots of kids rushing around the large rectangular rink. All of the boys and girls had rosy cheeks, and the sound of laughter and squeals of joy echoed in the open space. The blades scratched the ice as everyone cruised along: some fast, some slow, and some held onto the boards, terrified of falling. I was a decent skater and confident on the ice.

One weekend, I met a boy. His name was Chris, and he was very different from the boys in my class who hadn't hit puberty yet. Even though I was only ten, I had breasts, hips, and a heap of hormones I didn't know what to do with. Now, just because I had the curves and the appetite does not mean I actually looked like a teenager. Looking back at photos, it's quite evident I was a child in every other way—from the clothes to the awkwardness.

Chris left a huge impression on me; he was the first older boy to give me attention. He started chatting me up at the concession, and I was completely enticed. We hung around, and he told me he was sixteen and went to Dunbarton High School, where I would have attended if we had stayed in Pickering. I told him I was ten and in grade five, attending Valley Farm Public School. "You are so mature," he told me, "you look like you're in high school." This was music to my ears. Finally, someone saw I was beyond the maturity of my peers. I really viewed myself as a young woman and believed I was ready for the likes of my new friend.

Tall and heavyset with a short beard, Chris wasn't some-one I would have found attractive now, but as a young girl, this guy had my attention. It never crossed my mind that it was strange that this *much* older boy was talking to me. We exchanged numbers. My friend and I returned to our skating date and got picked up out front, as usual, by our parents. I tucked away my piece of paper with Chris' phone number written on it secretly in my pocket. Slipping away into daydreams about him, I imagined him as my boyfriend.

After a few phone calls, we made plans to meet at a nearby forest on Valley Farm Road. It was nearing the end of the school year, and the weather had warmed up. I wore heavy cotton shorts with a powder pink t-shirt with black polka dots. It was my favourite, and I wanted to look my best.

Chris and I met on the sidewalk that ran alongside the strip of forest. "Let's go in," he suggested, and I was happy to follow. We jumped over the guardrail separating the forest from the sidewalk and road. Hiking up the steep hill, we went deeper into the woods. The leaves crunched beneath our shoes on the forest floor, and low, thin branches scratched at my legs. At this point, I really had no clue what was about to happen. We started kissing, my first real kiss, but it's not with a boy: it's with a man. He asks me if I'm a virgin, and the words swirled around in my head while I tried to make sense of them.

I asked myself, *Has a virgin had sex? Or not? Which is it?* I had no clue what to say, so I guessed and said, "No." It was the wrong answer; I was absolutely a virgin. I had already had my first sexual experience through the assault the year before, but I still hadn't discovered sex.

He laid out his long leather coat on the cold forest ground and guided me onto it. Lying on my back feeling extremely vulnerable, he worked my favourite shorts off, along with my underwear. Then, he hovered on top of me, slowly trying to work his way inside me with his fingers first. I wanted to seem mature and pretended I knew what was going on, hiding my discomfort to his prodding. He took his hand away and positioned himself on top of me. Chris was heavy, and I felt so small underneath him as he tried to get his penis inside me. He got more aggressive, gyrating and pushing forward. I felt a ripping, burning sensation across my genitals, and I cried out in pain. Chris covered my mouth and shushed me while he continued to work. My tears ran down my face, and my thoughts raced. *Does a virgin have sex? Is it supposed to hurt this much? Why aren't I more ready? Is he my boyfriend now? If this is what he wants, I have to keep going so he will like me.* It reached a point where I couldn't tolerate the pain anymore, and I had become stiff as a board. I cried out, "Stop!" The next thing I remember was my long walk home. I wasn't too sure what had happened, but it sure didn't feel good. Why hadn't I been better at it? I didn't know that it would be so painful. *Is Chris my boyfriend now?*

I rushed straight to the bathroom, and when I pulled my shorts down, they were soaked in blood as if my period had come on full force. Still unsure of the reason, I felt incredibly embarrassed knowing I'd walked home with that huge stain on my shorts, on my heart, and down my cheeks from the tears I spilled. I shoved those shorts to the bottom of the hamper. I figured my Mom would think I had my period when she found them in the laundry. She never mentioned it to me.

It was a few weeks later when I finally saw Chris again. I had tried calling him a few times, but he was always busy. Finally, I ran into him at the rec, and he introduced me to a friend of his. I was a bit confused—I thought he had liked me. *Why does he want me to get to know his friend?* His friend invited me to go for a walk, and we wound up in a stairwell. He was really cute, and he smelled nice. We tossed off a few get-to-know-you questions, and it turned out that he was twenty-one! *Wow, I must be super mature for my age if both of these guys are into me.* I hadn't learned the word or definition of pedophile yet, and at that point, I didn't really understand anything about sex, anatomy, or boundaries.

"Have you ever given a blowjob?" he asked me.

I was honest that time and said, "No, I don't know what that is." He opened the zipper to his fitted jeans and pulled out a large, erect penis. Guiding my head down, he placed my mouth onto him and showed me the ropes.

"No teeth," he said. I had no clue what he meant, thinking I couldn't get rid of my teeth. He repeated the words a few more times, which I found really strange. I never saw either one of them again. I looked out for Chris and his friend on my future visits to the rec centre that year, but I figured they must have been really busy, and eventually, I moved on.

Harley was the next in line of many men to come, who took my tender heart and naivety and made a fool of me. Harley was sixteen, and he knew I was only ten. We met on my walk home from school one day. He invited me back to his place, which was only a five-minute walk from my home, and I was all in for more adventure, my heart full of the promise that this boy liked me.

We saw each other for a month or so. I went to his place after school and performed oral sex on him. The first time he ejaculated in my mouth, I was so shocked that I popped my head up, and it sprayed me in the eye, which stung so bad. This experience left me feeling very embarrassed while he just laughed at me, I felt like such an idiot. I didn't have a clue what I was doing, and I imagined he had been with much more experienced girls. *Not good enough.* These guys didn't continue to talk to me, which meant that I was not good enough. I needed more practice so I could have a boyfriend who loved me.

After having a few solid sexual experiences, my appetite started to grow. The other boys my age weren't capable of satisfying my curiosity, and honestly, I don't think they would have moved past first base. From this point on, I didn't look at a boy unless he was a few years older and ready to have sex.

I started having sexual encounters with my female friends to fill the times I didn't have a boyfriend and to meet my newly discovered needs. We dry humped each other's legs and even went as far as oral sex. I didn't enjoy it as much, but it was good practice in-between boyfriends.

Over the next year, I really started running wild. I hung out with a cousin who didn't live too far from me. She was a few years older, and her male friends were of great interest to me. One night, I didn't want to leave her place; I was feeling extremely rebellious against my parents and had significant anxiety about being around them. I finally broke down and told my cousin my secret about being molested when I was nine. It was a terrifying feeling, thinking that I was going to be in big trouble, even though I was trying to get out of trouble. I stayed the night and was driven straight to school the next day. They called me into the principal's office that morning. Terrified, I made my way down there. Two detectives waited for me in one of the offices, and they wanted to hear my story. I was mortified.

How was I supposed to tell two grown men my darkest, most shameful secret? I had never met them before, and they expected me to trust them. How could I bring myself to talk about the entire incident? Feeling so embarrassed, I left out the part when he rubbed my vagina. I felt the world betraying me as I sat with those detectives eyeing me. Judging me. The room felt as though it was closing in on us, and they kept questioning me, trying to get as much information as they could. With each passing minute, I got quieter and turned inside myself. My invisible walls went up. I did not answer any more questions.

My parents didn't handle it well. They allowed me to hide out in my room for the rest of my childhood. Police and Children's Aid both came to the conclusion that I was lying, and no charges were pressed. My parents' marriage, already rocky due to financial pressure, was breaking down, and they separated. It was time to move again.

Left feeling extremely lonely and isolated, I continued to remain invisible. I would sneak around the house to be as unseen as possible. Feelings of abandonment by my parents were strong. Even the two institutions put in place to protect me couldn't have cared less. The message that I was alone loomed over my existence like a dark cloud. *No one likes you.*

2

Scarborough

I was eleven years old when we moved to Scarborough, and we did not have a good start at our new location. One summer evening shortly after we had moved into our new house, my brother and I met up with a young lad a few years older. He came to our place in a car! He was only fourteen and said he'd been grounded by his parents; his response was to steal their car. Telling us not to worry, he knew how to drive and assured us it would be fun. It *was* fun! I had never been in a car without an adult before. We cruised around the Sheppard and Kingston area, music blaring and wheels screeching when he took a turn too fast. We had the windows down, and my long brown hair blew around wild and free. The lower half of my head was shaved, my first rebellion on my physical appearance.

As we sped around that evening, dusk fell upon us, and it seemed our new friend had no intention of returning home anytime soon. Then, we heard sirens wailing nearby. *Police!* Looking out the window from the backseat where I sat, I saw the red and blue flashing lights in the now dark sky. Fear took hold of my stomach, knowing we were going to be in trouble. The car's engine revved loudly, and we sped up; our friend was trying to get away! It was after nine—a few hours had passed so quickly. Additional sirens and lights appeared, and adrenaline pumped through my body. I was terrified of getting caught but thrilled by the excitement of it all. The police cornered us, but our friend took one more chance at getting away. He pulled into the parking lot of a new condo development and off-roaded through a field on the property. The car slammed up and down on the uneven grass and dirt, jostling us around inside. The police cars swarmed us, and eventually, the car couldn't handle the uneven ground, and he finally gave up. The vehicle came to a stop, and there was a red and blue lightshow outside. I couldn't tell how many police cars were out there, but we were surrounded.

"Come out with your hands up!" an officer shouted many times through an amplifier. It was just like Cops on TV, a show I had watched dozens of times. Each of us opened our own door to start making our way out of the car. We were greeted by a dozen cops with their guns pointing right at us. Many voices yell, "Get down on the ground!" at us, and we immediately obeyed.

They handcuffed me and put me into the back of a cop car alone. This was my third interaction with the police in the past year. The first was after telling the truth about my first sexual assault; the second was when I had been accurately accused of stealing money from the girl's change room at basketball camp.

When we arrived at the police station, they interviewed my brother and me separately. As I sat and waited my turn, I wondered what was going to happen. Would they strip-search me? Take my fingerprints? Would I have to spend the night in a cell? I looked around the building and noticed it was very brightly lit and had a few interview rooms but was otherwise an open space with desks. *Where are the other criminals?* I thought. I really didn't have any information to give them. We had just moved into town, and I barely knew this kid. My interrogation was quick—I said, "I don't know" often. The only information I gave them was my name and address and that I had just met this kid a few days ago. I had never met his parents, didn't know where he went to school, and never saw him again after this incident.

I don't remember my mom picking us up from the police station. She usually wasn't as mad at me when I got into trouble alongside my brother, who rarely got into mischief. It was almost like if he was involved, it must have been reasonable trouble to get into. I always felt we were treated very differently, but this time, I was happy we were in it together as I'm sure it saved me from harsher punishment.

My parents separated before we moved to Scarborough, and this was one of the reasons we moved. We couldn't afford the house in Pickering anymore as interest rates on mortgages had skyrocketed, and it was now just going to be my mother, brother, and I living together. Once again, I had to start at another new school, though this time seemed like the most comfortable adjustment. My precocious puberty made me look like a teenage girl now, and this definitely gave me a commanding presence.

I ended up making really good friends in the grade eight class above me, so I finally caught a break in the social standings. We met at recess and after school, and soon, we hung out all weekend. I was so happy to belong to a crew. A couple of the girls had older sisters, and this became my introduction to cigarettes and alcohol.

During Christmas break that year, my mom, brother, and I travelled to Nova Scotia to spend Christmas with my grandparents. It was an adventure, to say the least. We almost got killed when a transport truck sideswiped us on a highway in Quebec during a whiteout snowstorm. Our car spun in circles right into the guardrail. My mom gathered herself quickly and drove us off the highway to make sure we were okay. We had all been whipped around but had no visible damage. My mom was terrified to drive the rest of the way, but she got us there.

I was so happy we were spending Christmas with family, as we didn't really have any in Ontario. Christmas morning was excellent - lots of gifts and a pleasant time spent with family. I felt so safe at my grandma's house, and she was one of my favourite people. In the afternoon on Christmas Day, I ran into my grumpy grandpa at the bottom of the stairs. The house they lived in was over eighty years old, and everything was sectioned off with doors leading into every room, including the kitchen. He cornered me against a wall, grabbed my face with his two bear paw hands, and landed a wet, disgusting French kiss on me. I could not believe my grandfather had his tongue in my mouth. I was horrified and shocked, and I'm sure he saw it on my face. He pulled back and burst out laughing in a god-awful cackle that anyone who knows him knows what it sounded like. He had a laugh that said, "Screw you, and you, and screw you too." I never spoke a word of it to anyone and tucked it away inside with all of my other sorrows.

By the age of twelve, I smoked every day and drank on the weekends. I often stole liquor and money from my parents. My dad had eventually moved back home after having a serious accident at work. Falling from a roof and breaking both arms and multiple ribs, he also had a severe concussion. He needed us to take care of him because he could hardly do anything for himself. Down to one income, my parents were under extreme financial pressure at this time.

I met some more of the older kids in the neighbourhood and finally had a boyfriend. His name was Devon, and he was a nineteen-year-old black man. He was six feet tall and must have weighed over 200 pounds, husky with a bit of a beer belly. Devon was always happy, and he had a beautiful smile and a soft voice. He was really kind to me, and I looked forward to seeing him after school and on weekends. Of course, my parents had no clue about Devon. Though I never saw drugs or guns on him, one of the other older girls told me he sold marijuana and carried a gun. It didn't faze me, however. In my eyes, he was like a giant teddy bear; I couldn't imagine him hurting anyone. After a few weeks of hooking up at the park near my school with other friends, we drove to his apartment in his old four-door Honda sedan to have sex. He lived in the projects on Tuxedo Court, still in Scarborough, just a less desirable part. I had never been to low-income housing before.

My first time there, we went straight to his room to have sex. We lay on a queen size bed with navy blue sheets. He climbed on top of me and had his way. I scanned the room while he groaned and gyrated. After he had finished with his orgasm, we lay in bed smoking cigarettes, and I saw a small black creature scurry across the floor.

What the fuck was that? I wonder. A cockroach? Feeling very uneasy, I couldn't wait to leave. I headed to the bathroom to pee and surveyed my surroundings very carefully to ensure I didn't have a run-in with one of those nasty bugs. While I was in the bathroom, one scurried out from behind the toilet, and I let out a little scream. It was huge! He laughed at me as we got dressed, saying they wouldn't harm me. I couldn't get back into the car fast enough. He always dropped me off at the school near my house, and I walked home so my parents didn't catch us together.

A few days or weeks after we started having sex, I noticed a foul odor every time I used the bathroom. A few days later,

I saw a creamy white substance in my underwear, and I felt uncomfortable down there. I told my mom something was wrong, and she took me to see our family doctor. The doctor ran a few tests and came back with a solemn look on his face. He told us both I had an STD. I was shocked because I didn't really know about that kind of thing yet, and they were shocked because I was twelve and they couldn't believe I was already having sex.

"With who?" they asked. I told them a half-story about a boy I had been seeing who was only a few years older because I knew better than to supply too many details. To ease their concern and hopefully de-escalate the situation, I told them the boy and I had broken it off. The doctor was very concerned about me getting pregnant and recommended we consider birth control. He asked me to tell my mom if I decided to have sex again.

We never spoke about this again. I wasn't grilled for hours to find out who this boy really was or when I had lost my virginity. My mother quickly swept it under our dusty rug, which gave me the impression that what I was doing, though unfavourable, was okay. I believed the doctor when he said it was a good idea for me to protect myself from pregnancy and decided that, yes, I should start birth control. My mother and I didn't communicate about anything other than chores and curfew, so I thought it best to write her a note. Nervously, I printed out a note on a small piece of paper.

Dear Mom,

I have met a boy that I really like. We may start having sex. Please get me some birth control. Thanks.

Love,
Deirdre

I slipped it into her jewellery box and awaited a response. Days passed, and my mother didn't approach me. I decide to peek into the jewellery box to see if she had found the note. When I opened it up, the note was gone. Yes, she had found the note, and maybe she was going to leave the birth control in my room once she acquired it, and we wouldn't have to talk about it at all. Weeks passed; I came to the conclusion that she was not going to help me. *Maybe it isn't as important as the doctor made it seem*, I thought. Looking back now, as a mother of a twenty-year-old daughter, I'm floored my mother hadn't gone to the police. Twelve was *way* too young to be making these choices, and I would have wanted to find out my daughter hadn't been coerced into having sex. I imagined my mother opening her jewellery box and seeing the note I'd left her, feeling fear, anxiety, and shame rush up inside of her at the realization that her little girl was living a life far beyond her years.

A week or two later, Devon, the teddy bear, and I headed out to a dance hall party to pick up or drop something off to his older brother who was a promoter of those types of events. Devon seemed to know the bouncers, so we bypassed security and headed into the club. Reggae music blared, and I was one of the only white people in the room—and the only twelve-year-old. Looking around in amazement, it looked like a big concert. I'd never been to one but had seen them in music videos and movies. Everyone danced, smoke filled the air, and I felt really out of place, but my fear was surprisingly low. Devon held my hand tight like I was his possession, and I knew I was safe with him.

I met his older brother for the first time that night. Devon introduced him as Dwight, then left me with him and said he would be right back. Dwight didn't look like Devon at all. He was even a bit taller but slender and very lean. His skin was a bit darker, and I found him attractive. We chatted a bit, and I saw by the way his eyes sized me up that he was attracted to me. He passed me his number and said I should give him a call sometime. I tucked it away in my pocket with a little smile on my face and thought, *Wow, I'm so grown up. Look at these men all over me.* How easy it was for them to prey on the young.

As soon as Devon came back to get me, we left the party. It probably wasn't his jam, or maybe having sex was higher on his list of things he liked to do. That wasn't the last time I saw his brother. I called Dwight, being super curious as to what he was all about. I was looking for attention and entertainment at all times, and Devon was unavailable.

Dwight came to pick me up and started driving to his house. *Oh god,* I thought, *please don't let Devon be there.* I suddenly felt a bit afraid of being caught by my boyfriend with his brother. To my relief, no one was home.

We had sex, smoked, and then made our way back to my end of Scarborough. Seeing him only the one time, a quick fix seemed to suit us both fine. Things between Devon and I dwindled off after that. I wasn't sad to have lost the connection with him, though I felt an urge to find a replacement quickly.

I continued to party on the weekends and steal money from my mom for cigarettes and McDonalds. I was suspended for smoking on school property and snuck out after curfew. Starting to lie about my sleepovers at friends' houses, I stayed out all night, and I drank in parks or back allies. Eventually, I found a new Devon; we met at a subway station. His name was David, he was a black man, and very kind. He was only a bit taller than me, slim, rode a skateboard, and was over 25. He invited me over to his place because he lived on his own, and I was up for the adventure. We had a lot of sex, multiple times per visit. On one of our visits, I decided to stay overnight, not wanting the party to end. The next day, I decided to call home to let my parents know I would be home the following day. I wanted to be out the entire weekend; I really enjoyed the freedom and did not adhere well to anyone trying to enforce rules upon me. Instead, they demanded I come home right away. I hung up the phone and didn't plan on following their instructions. A few minutes later, David's phone rang. We looked at each other with an "oh fuck" expression as he answered the phone.

David: "Hello?"
Dad: "This is Constable John McKinnon. We have information that Deirdre is staying at your place. She needs to be sent home right away, or we will be coming by to get her."
David: "Yes, sir, she's on her way."

David hung up the phone, looked at me, and said, "I'm pretty sure that was your dad pretending to be a cop. Time for you to go—I can't have the police here." Of course, I agreed—I didn't want to deal with cops either. David walked me to the subway and off I went, wondering what punishment awaited me—surely more rules to break.

I look back on that time and wonder what my parents thought. Why didn't they call the cops? I was clearly at a grown man's place: what story were they telling themselves to make this okay? I believe they were still traumatized by the police visit back when I was eleven, and they didn't want anything to do with that kind of *help* either. David and I kept in occasional contact during that year, hooking up every once in a while. It was a hard year; I was always in trouble, though I still managed to keep my grades up and excelled in English, story writing, and speeches.

There were glaring signs that I was about to turn a corner into further unknown territory; I was continually breaking boundaries and fuelling myself with cigarettes and alcohol.

Depression was definitely already very present. I was still isolating myself at home from the rest of my family. Anger and insecurity boiled inside of me, and I didn't understand it. There was a deep knowing that I didn't belong. I was ignored at home and I felt like an underdog in my social circle, always being the youngest and feeling like I didn't have much to offer.

Pulling all of our medications out of the cupboard one day, I thought about downing them all to stop the pain I felt. I lined up Tylenol, Advil, allergy meds, and a few unknown prescriptions. After contemplating it for fifteen minutes or so, I wondered, *What will happen? What if I don't die right away? What if I am left in a tremendous amount of physical pain? What if I die? What's on the other side?* Fear of the unknown stopped me from doing anything that day, and I tucked all of the pills back in the cupboard.

Sex and alcohol would have to mask this broken girl for now.

3

Addicted

I vividly remember standing outside of a Pizza Hut Delivery in 1992. It was a tiny plaza on John Street in Thornhill that also hosted a convenience store. That summer, we had moved from Scarborough. I was stuck spending July and August alone and bored, dreading the upcoming school year and the thought of trying to fit in with another new class of kids. My brother and I barely spoke at the time, and I felt like the black sheep in the family.

In the dead of summer, I wore maroon Doc Martens, flared jeans, and a baggy t-shirt, a cross between an alternative reggae/hip hop style. I would soon learn that this was the opposite of how my new, mostly Jewish, classmates dressed. On the first day of grade eight, I stood out like a drag queen at a line-dancing gig. If only I'd had the same confidence the dancing queen did. Now, you would think that my fashion choices would have saved me from being preyed on by horny men, but apparently, a lot of them don't judge those choices.

The pizza delivery guy passed me a few times throughout the day and occasionally stopped to have a smoke with me. He was handsome and bi-racial, which was in line with my type at the time. Quite a bit older than I should have been looking at, but did I mention I was bored and lonely? I don't remember his name, but the age will never disappear from memory—thirty-five! It stayed with me because he was the oldest man to come on to me knowing my age, which was twelve at the time. I remember feeling special, wanted; I'd found an adult who wanted to spend time with me. We made plans to meet after his shift one evening. He picked me up, and we headed to his place in Scarborough, a small and pathetic apartment. We started having sex, and I was swept into the lure of being desired, again. I don't remember seeing him again after that night; maybe remorse kicked in for him after the climax of pleasure had lifted. These flings filled me up, then tore me down. I was desperate to find love, even at the cost of my self-respect. By this age, I understood that what I was doing was wrong, but the lure to possible love was too strong.

The rest of the summer was a wash, and the start of grade eight came with a deeper depression. I showed up wearing my Scarborough styles, Malcolm X gear and all. It was evident to me immediately that I was an outsider. The other kids tried to be friendly and ask questions, but I felt as though I'd landed in a foreign country. I talked different, dressed odd, and listened to entirely different music. Surely, these kids had never listened to reggae and clearly hadn't been to a dance-hall party.

I just couldn't make a connection with anyone; my communication skills were extremely poor, and I felt like I needed to hide everything about myself. Feeling like an outcast, I knew it was the beginning of a very long road paved by shame, anger, and insecurity. I dreaded going to school every day and felt a great deal of stress, trying to cope with my misplacement in life. Having no relationship with my parents at this point was hard; they were useless in helping me find my way. It seemed to be too late anyhow; I was already set on this trajectory, fuelled by the lies and poison of men I'd met along the way.

After a month or so, I finally made a friend. Her name was Mandy, and we got through the rest of the year together. We were two misfits suffering similar exile, and at that point, I didn't care that she was a loner. I was just so tired of being alone myself. Funny enough, by the end of the year, the Scarborough fashion had made its way up to Thornhill, and at least the boys were starting to dress like me. The music made its way as well, and by the time we are on our year-end school trip, we were all rapping our way from Toronto to Quebec.

Graduation came with pride. I was so happy to finally leave elementary school behind and move on to high school, where I assumed my peeps were. I had a boyfriend, Myles, an eighteen-year-old man who was totally cool with dating a kid. He wasn't my perfect type—not enough rough edges—but he had a car and he wanted to have lots of sex, so I kept him around. Sex had become a drug for me. I craved its familiarity. It was the one thing I knew I was good at; I needed it to make me feel special, accepted, and, most importantly, loved. I equated sex with love. In my mind, if we were fucking, it meant you loved me, even if it was only for the moment.

My mom and I went shopping for my graduation dress together. I never, *ever* wore dresses, skirts, or anything feminine. We finally both agreed on something long and airy in navy blue with tiny white flowers. I wore this dress out after the ceremony with my classmates to see my boyfriend and came home with it ruined. It was dirty from lying in grass and dirt outside while we fucked, ripped by his aggressive, lusting hands.

Anger lit my mother's face when she saw the dress in tatters. It was a perfect show of how I took anything nice and ruined it instantly. Moments, memories, and even clothes. Nothing had meaning to me other than getting my fix.

My home life was quiet; I spent all of my time holed away in my room, listening to music. I had a large butcher knife hidden under my mattress at that time: it protected me from the possibilities of abuse, which I seemed to find everywhere.

My parents left me alone; communication was never something I was taught and I struggled over the years to figure it out. I liked the lack of it at the time, because as a teen, it allowed me to hide all of the shitty things I was doing. Feeling positive my parents were extremely embarrassed of me, I had wished I never existed too. Self-loathing every time I was alone, often crying myself to sleep, comforted only by the sharp, shiny knife that lay parallel beneath me.

The summer leading into grade nine was the last time they sent me to my grandmother's in Nova Scotia. I spent an entire month with her in the quiet country. My grandmother was the best; we sat out on her porch and smoked cigarettes in the evening. She told me stories of her troubled younger years, and I felt a real kinship to her. Gram was the one person who I felt loved me unconditionally.

I had a friend across the street from years before, but her mother had decided I was too much of a city girl and wasn't a positive influence on her precious little girl. We were pen-pals, and my letters of boys and adventure were what had revealed my bad influence. Clearly, her mother had made the right decision.

Even in the tiny town of Milford, I'd found myself someone to fuck. I met him at the ice cream shop, and we headed over to the school. He cruised around on his skateboard, and I walked, forever pulling up my baggy pants that were ripped at the hem from always stepping on them. We found a nook at the nearby school to hide in and stood up doggystyle to do the deed. A few minutes of pleasure, and I never saw him again. I got my fix.

A few days later, I flew home, and I was so excited to see the boyfriend I had to leave behind for a whole month. We lasted a week or two, hooked up for sex a few times, and then he ended it. I wasn't too heartbroken over this one; he was a little tame for my taste anyway.

High school started up, and it was time to begin a new chapter. I had to start over in the friend's department, which was horrible, but I managed to find some misfits to blend in with. Trouble finds trouble, and then it breeds more trouble.

Here came my introduction to drugs. Marijuana, mushrooms, LSD, and hash were on the menu at my new school, and I liked it. They were just as good as sex. Now I had more medication to either help me feel or not feel, depending on what I needed.

Skipping class to get high started immediately, and it wasn't long before I was on a daily excursion to the principal's office. I failed all of my classes, and my mom began dropping me off at school because I couldn't be trusted to get there on the bus. The more school I missed, the more terrified I was to attend. I knew I was falling behind, and the thought of catching up felt daunting. More drugs to forget, to hide from reality. I was falling deeper into my depression, and the only thing that made me happy was sex and drugs.

I got into a new party scene on the weekends. Raving. It was amazing. New underground EDM music, secret locations we arrived at after catching a school bus that left Nathan Phillips Square in Toronto at 10 pm on Saturdays. My friends and I started using molly, a drug that made me feel warm, fuzzy, loved, and happy. Everything I wasn't capable of feeling while I was sober. It was magical; the drug made me dance and feel all night long. Everyone at the party was a lost soul, arriving to make peace with the week or life they've had. We were all one, vibrating together, understanding one another; it felt safe, like a tribe.

I needed more money to keep up with the costs of these parties and the drugs. I was earning $20 per week for allowance, and I cleaned the entire house for this money. But the weekends cost me at least $40, so I started stealing and panhandling on the streets of Toronto to make up for the lack of cash.

The more I partied, the more addicted I became. I quickly started spending Friday to Sunday in Toronto, staying at strangers' places or on the streets if I didn't hook up with anyone. I'd ridden the subway and bus system hundreds of times trying to stay warm and/or dry, or just to have a safe place to lay my head. Though I never stepped foot into a shelter. I didn't want help; the reason I was out there was to escape, forget, and feel free from responsibility. It never crossed my mind to look for help. I thought the sex and drugs were doing a fine job at keeping me together; who needs adulting anyway?

I didn't attend the second semester of grade nine at all, and I failed seven out of eight courses that year. Somehow, I still managed to pick up a math credit. At that point, my parents didn't know what to do with me. When they tried to enforce rules, I packed a bag and left for days on end. I hooked up with the friends I made in the rave scene and partied all of the pain away.

After one of these absences, I came home to pick up some fresh clothes. I was with my temporary boyfriend, Colin, at the time. At this time, I was fourteen, and he was in his twenties. There were plenty of these men out there ready and willing to take advantage of a child. He was extremely immature, homeless, and a full-blown drug addict. Colin waited for me at the nearby park while I approached the house. Shit, my dad was home and working in the garden. He asked what I was doing there, and I replied that I was coming for clothes. He wouldn't allow me to come in the house. I said, "Fuck you." He punched me in the face, and I dropped to the ground.

"You're not welcome here," he said. I felt my insides slump, and I told myself that I never was.

I took off to my friend's house down the street and called my mom in tears. She didn't know what to do with me. "Please come home, let's figure things out," she said. I told her I would come home the following day and meet her. I did, and I promised her I would change. As usual, my parents were full of anger and fear. They wanted nothing to do with me, but I was only fourteen—they couldn't just let me be. I made decisions for myself as if I were twenty, and it took a toll on everyone.

Colin introduced me to heroin. We partied on molly and crystal meth all the time, and that shit got me wired. Jaw grinding, teeth clenching, paranoid about everything, and suspicious of everyone. That feeling of love, joy, and connection to my peeps was long gone. Doses doubled and tripled to find that feeling again, and I felt desperate to replicate it. When the drugs first kicked in, I got a glimpse of the elated feeling I longed for, and then the chase was on. After a few days and nights of this, we tried something else to help us come down and release us from the black hole we were stuck in.

Colin called a friend from a payphone, and off we went to hook up with him. We met at a park in the early morning, and I took my first hit of the smoke streaming off of tinfoil through a rolled-up bill. A feeling of heaviness washed over me, and my mind slowed down. Complete sedation. It also came with huge waves of nausea, and I puked in public. I had no self-awareness, so that didn't bother me at all. The beautiful sun, people milling around, and all the other signs of life happening around us were too much to handle in that state. A tai chi class gathered on a grassy area twenty feet away from us with what looked like fifty participants attending. The grass was a perfect shade of green, and everything was well-manicured. A few homeless people took up space around the park, along with the odd dog walker and a few joggers. Life was in full throttle for them and slowing right the fuck down for me. I wanted to be somewhere I could really disappear; the park in the bustle of the morning was just too alive.

We headed back to this guy's apartment to continue our attempt at disappearing into a drug-induced stupor. We took the bus, and I slipped in and out of awareness. We arrived at his pad—unwelcoming, a real hole in the wall, and the filthiest place I've ever been in. Garbage sat in piles everywhere, dirty dishes covered the counters in heaps, and the smell of old urine permeated through what looked like an indoor garbage alley. I felt so uncomfortable; I barely knew my boyfriend, and this was my first time meeting his friend. We barely communicated with each other because we were so high and delirious.

We did a few more hits, and I felt completely lost in a time warp. All of the windows were covered, and it was dark, making it impossible to know if it was day or night.

We made a bed out of sleeping bags right in the middle of the kitchen floor, where I had one of the deepest sleeps ever. I eventually woke up to use the bathroom and peeked out from the covers I hid under. Garbage and food containers littered my visual survey from the kitchen to the bathroom. I listened carefully to hear if anyone else was up. It was dead quiet, so I dug myself out to take a pee. My bladder felt like it was ready to burst, and I had no clue what time it was. I sat on the disgusting toilet seat because I felt too weak to squat over it. Burning pain while the flow got started quickly replaced the feeling of great relief. There was no toilet paper, so I drip-dried. I noticed my underwear was in rough shape.

Days of bodily fluids started to build up a crusty layer, but I didn't have an extra pair. I slid them back on, and I quietly slipped back onto the makeshift bed. I caught sight of a clock—3 a.m. or p.m.? Fuck it—sleep called out to me, and all I wanted to do was disappear into it.

The next time I woke, I found myself alone; Colin and his friend had left. Honestly, I felt relieved to be by myself. The depression and self-loathing after a bender like that were best spent on my own. I took a quick look around to find some change for the bus. No coins—brutal. Taking a huge swig from a bottle containing warm, flat mountain dew, it reminded me I hadn't brushed my teeth in days. I ran my tongue over the fuzz on my teeth and had the first urge in days to go home. Home. My parents were going to be pissed.

The clock said 4:30, and upon opening the door to sunshine, I knew it was late afternoon. I had done the walk of shame so many times before; dirty and used, I took the first steps. Closing the door, I re-entered the world and left behind the filth and broken dreams on the other side of the door.

Squinting my eyes to protect them from the awful sun and thinking, *How can the sun shine when I'm this miserable?* It was a reminder to myself that what I was doing with my life was wrong. If I hated the sun, there was a serious problem at hand.

I picked a direction and started walking; I had no clue where I was. The street names did not ring any bells. *Keep walking; find a subway station or a payphone.* With my head down and feet dragging, I finally found a payphone. I grabbed the receiver and pressed 0 to send a collect call to my parents. My mom answered with a voice full of concern.

"Where are you?" she gushed. I gave her my coordinates, and they told me to sit tight and that she would arrive in an hour. As the car pulled up, I felt a great sense of relief. I picked myself up off the sidewalk, and I slid into the back and waited for the attack of questions. I couldn't bear the thought of panhandling in this condition to earn money to get myself home; telling them a bit of the story seemed like a better choice. I told them it wasn't a big deal; I was only away for a few days; I lost track of time having fun with my friends, but everything was ok. In my mind, I had been gone for four nights. It was Sunday, right?

My parents told me it was Wednesday, making it a full week since I'd last been home or spoken to them. Wednesday? *How did three days disappear on me? What else don't I remember?* My mind was still blurry, and I passed out again until we arrived home.

I stayed with my parents for a few days to recover, sleep, eat, and shower. Then, I put a bit of money together to head downtown for the weekend again. And again and again.

4

Escorting

In 1995, we moved to Richmond Hill. My parents were finally starting to recover from the massive financial hit they took in 1991. My dad had recovered from his accident and was in college to follow a new career path. They hoped for a fresh start, but we only moved about ten kilometres from where we were in Thornhill, and I still had close contact with all of my friends.

I started at a new high school, Alexander Mackenzie, to repeat grade nine. Though I was not looking forward to another year of trying to fit in, I was still willing to give it a go. At fifteen I was covered in piercings and thought I looked great. I had both sides of my nose done at this point, a stud on one side and a ring on the other. Later, I had removed the two nose piercings and replaced them with a ring through my septum, otherwise known as a bull ring. I also had a side lip ring. Each time I came home with a new piercing, I felt my mother's wrath of fury and shame. She despised my fashion choices; I was wearing gigantic baggy jeans and t-shirts with aliens on them. I had cute baby backpacks for my weekend adventures downtown. My choice in hairstyles was still off the norm, and at this time, I had my entire head shaved and bleached blonde. I stood out like a sore thumb at school and kept to myself for the most part. After a few weeks, I made friends with a girl I would nickname Friffin as a play on her last name. She was totally weird, had hair coloured like the rainbow, and smoked lots of pot. She was also repeating grade nine, and we got along just fine.

It wasn't long before we skipped classes together and got stoned out of our minds. We extended our crew to a few others over those months to include Elisha, Dalton, and Jordy. We all met at lunch or after school to get high. On the weekends, I was either downtown raving, hanging with my old crew in Thornhill, or spending time at Friffin's.

Eventually, Jordy invited me over to her place one weekend, and I was thrilled. I really looked up to her. She was a year older, had a good name for herself at the school, and was a stoner as well. We got high on weed, hash, and mushrooms and settled into her bed to enjoy the trip and watch *Natural Born Killers*. We cuddled up pretty close to one another, but I did not think much of it until she brushed her arm against me in a way that I totally understood. *She's hitting on me?* I had not pegged her as bisexual or even curious. *Ok, I'm down.* We fooled around, and it was glorious. I had been with a few girls already and had always been the pursuer. This was the first time a girl has come on to me, and I was in heaven. After this encounter, we were inseparable. We hooked up at school on break, weekends, after school—any free time we had, we spent it together.

Jordy's mom terrified me. She was the type of woman who said what was on her mind—no filter. She had no issue looking me up and down for assessment with a suspicious eye. She was right to be suspicious. Even though I felt a bit uncomfortable with how forward she was, I always felt welcome and safe in her home. I also wanted to be with Jordy as often as possible, so it was a necessity. Jordy and I slept over at each other's houses on the weekends, and we were a really great pair. We took care of each other as best we could—two broken girls trying to make sense out of life. Each of us carried so much pain, but there was always acceptance and understanding between us as to why we were each *so fucked up*!

Jordy was a petite girl at only 5'3" and 115 pounds, and she had beautiful brown hair that hit her waist and a few blonde highlights. She had a sparkle in her eye that drew me in, an invitation that was like a drug itself. Her mischievous smile held secrets that made my heart rate increase, ready for the excitement that time with her entailed. She had amazing breasts and athletic ability, although that part of her had started to slip as the drugs took their place.

Jordy created a map of her suffering through cutting. This was my first experience with this behaviour. Though she had cuts on her stomach and inner thighs, her arms showed the worst of it. My heart always broke when a new wound appeared. I knew her pain was deep, and she struggled to express it. The only coping we understood was to get high.

We mostly did molly, acid, mushrooms, and occasionally crystal meth, though neither of us liked it that much. I always felt very safe with Jordy; there was a great sense she cared about me, and I could depend on her to have my back. This familiar feeling between us forged a lifelong friendship with many highs and lows, ins and outs.

At school, I failed my first semester again, and they put me in a special program in a small classroom with all the other misfits who were struggling. I will never forget the teacher, Mrs. Faulkner. She understood the difficulties kids like me experienced and really made an effort to help. The school didn't want to keep me there as I was truant most of the time, and eventually, they shipped me off to Bayview Secondary School for a new program starting there with Mrs. Faulkner. I attended class enough to get my third math credit for grades nine through eleven and then dropped out of school forever.

Jordy and I drifted in and out of a relationship, moving on to other lovers but always remaining friends until the introduction of a man named Pat. This guy embodied the perfect image of white trash. He must have been in his thirties, and he had a shaved head, bleach blonde cut-off skin-tight jeans made into shorts, a band t-shirt, and a pock-marked face to boot. Jordy invited me over to his buddy's place—a garage turned into a bachelor pad. These guys were into tattooing and had a machine and some ink with them. Of course, I jumped at the chance to get a free tattoo. I decided I would like stick-figures, alternating boy/girl to form an anklet. We started with a boy in blue, and I was immediately in severe pain, so I decided I did not like tattooing! We'd already started, and I really wanted one, so I kept moving forward. Next up came the girl in pink. And that's where it stopped; I could not handle the discomfort, so he left me left with a stick-figure boy and girl holding hands on my ankle. Thankfully, I did not go through with the rest, and the image faded over time, now barely visible.

Jordy fucked Pat, which meant I wanted to. We were very competitive with each other at times, and this ended up causing many fights. We took turns grabbing his attention until I met Kathy. Our first introduction was at a house party one weekend in Richmond Hill, where I went to meet Pat. I knew a few other people there, and I had a few drinks and smoked some weed. Kathy was tall with beautiful, long dancer's legs, making her extremely fit and eye-catching. I knew she had already met Jordy, and I knew I needed to sleep with her. I'm not sure if they were already dating, but at the time, this wasn't an issue. We found an empty bedroom to make out in, and I slipped her clothes off without a fight. She was ready to play, and I was all in. Kathy and I remained friends for years, and we dated for a short period of time, but she was very insecure, and it was even too much for me.

Kathy's first girlfriend was connected to a good friend of mine, Lina. She lived in the same building as Friffin, and we often hung out after school or on weekends. When I turned sixteen in 1996, Lina hooked me up with someone who worked as a bouncer at the local strip club, Fantasia, for a job as a cashier. I guess they were desperate for workers and had no issue with underage girls.

At Fantasia, I worked as a cashier in one of the private back rooms. I wore black pants and a white blouse, dressed as though I could have been a hostess or server in a fancy restaurant. I had day hours, 11–4, and the club was usually dead during these times. Occasionally, I took an evening shift, and that was always action-packed. My conservative outfit helped me blend into the background, and I was perfectly fine with that. My code name at work was Juliette-Two, and I listened on a headpiece for the heads up that undercover police entered the club. If that were ever the case, I was to head into the private room to let the dancers know they needed to keep all dances above board. This meant no hand jobs, blow jobs, or sex, which were all common extras in the strip club scene at the time.

This was my first real job with a paycheque. It helped me continue on my path of self-destruction, sex, drugs, and self-loathing. I hooked up with different guys every weekend; as long as they provided the party supplies, I supplied the fun in the form of sex. By now, those memories have faded, but I do remember the extreme highs of the drugs and the feelings of acceptance gained by giving my body to anyone who fit the criteria. I also remember the extreme lows when the drugs ran out, and I felt worthless for giving away little pieces of myself with each sex act I performed.

I was introduced to escorting through Jordy in 1997. It was a few months shy of my seventeenth birthday. We eventually made up over our silly Pat dispute and were both big into partying. Our tastes became more and more expensive. Cocaine made its grand entrance up my nose and took me to a state of oblivion I loved. It was an expensive habit, but my girl and I hadn't planned on kicking it any time soon.

She made friends with some sleazy woman named Ziola who paid Jordy to roleplay and be her sub in S&M while feeding her new addiction. Ziola set us up an interview to get us into prostituting to help us make more money, and we were all in. The two of us met her friend and his buddy. We showed up to the condo, ready and assuming we were going fuck them. I was surprised when they led us into a bedroom that had dildos on the bed and told us to "have fun" before closing the door and leaving us on our own.

The two of us climbed onto the bed. I looked around wondering how they were possibly going to know what we were doing and what we were capable of. *Cameras? Are they out in the living room watching us?* It was totally fucking creepy. These guys were in their fifties, I was only sixteen, and Jordy was seventeen. We looked at each other, smiling, and I thought, *God, this is easy. All you need me to do is fuck around with my girl like I usually do?* We happily did what they wanted us to.

I told them I was only sixteen. "Isn't it illegal?" I asked.

"Don't worry—as long as you always say you're eighteen, there will be no problem. I need a fake name and your measurements," the guy in charge said.

This was very exciting to me, making up a false identity. I felt so grown up and in control of my life. Alexus! That was going to be my working girl name. 34B (which they advertised as a C) 26, 34. Blonde, green eyes, eighteen years old.

He also invited us to live with him and his girlfriend. We rented the spare bedroom in their Scarborough condo, which was also the call centre. His girlfriend booked the calls, pretending with each one she was the girl the customer was calling about. Carrie must have been in her thirties and was extremely overweight. She had long blonde hair with a mis-shapen ponytail and wore tights with a sloppy t-shirt every day. There was food being delivered to her constantly. Looking back, I realized she was stuffing away her feelings with food.

The condo was off of Highway 401, just east of Toronto, and overlooked the Scarborough Town Centre. We had a small room, but it had a double bed and a private bathroom. Living together made us so happy. We brought our clothes, CDs and even a few stuffed animals. I couldn't believe how lucky we were to find this awesome set-up where we could be together, make good money, and disappear from a life I hated. We finally had a safe and quiet spot to binge out on cocaine. So many days were spent afterward holding each other as we quietly prayed to fall asleep, to end the suffering that came with the last line. We felt an ache, a yearning to do more. It felt as though someone had died, and we were mourning the loss. With daylight peering through the curtains and the sweet melodies of our music playing, sleep would eventually rescue us until we had to get back to work. Living at the call centre was great; I would wake up, shower, throw on my make-up, and be ready to roll out. A driver met us outside in the lobby and took us to our calls. We had a decent split of the money. All I needed was enough to get a pack of smokes, some coke, and a meal. That was my life—all about the drugs. The more escorting I did, the more coke I did, and it became a vicious cycle.

I don't really remember many of the men I saw; it was mostly routine. The ones who stand out were the ones who made me feel extremely uncomfortable. One time, I went to the superintendent of an old beat-up building. Upon walking into his apartment, I was disturbed by the smell and by him. He wore jeans and a stained white wife-beater tank top. His belly hung out over his pants. He was short and balding; he had a few wispy hairs on his head, reminding me of a baby. I made my standard phone call into the agency to confirm I had received payment, then they would let the driver know.

Time to get down to business. We walked into his bedroom, and he got situated on his bed. Looking around, I was shocked by all of the junk; this guy was a total packrat. I focused on him, and he smiled with a mouth that was missing a lot of teeth. *God, what do I do? Can I back out of a call? Shit, I need the money!* I zoned out, planning to finish as quick as possible and get the fuck out of there. When I pulled out a condom and rolled it onto his small penis, I wished I was somewhere else. Mentally, I allowed myself to disappear. I tried to make his sickly smell fade away. Closing my eyes, I headed off into another world while Alexus took over to get the job done.

After we finished, I called the agency, and they sent the driver over. I headed outside, lit up a smoke, and shook off the creepy feeling left over. Hopping into the back of the car, I made small talk with the driver while I finished my smoke. The rest of the night, I stayed quiet and looked out the window to watch the neighbourhoods fly by.

The city looked gloomy in the winter when all the snow piled up along the side of the road and turned brown from the pollution and dirt kicked up by the traffic. At that point in my life, I felt completely numb. I had no feelings inside, and my physical self was only an empty vessel carrying around my shallow soul. All I cared about was getting my calls done for the day so I could buy the drugs to get me high and wash away all of my pain and insecurities. Like the fresh snowfall covered up the unattractive mess on the road beneath the car on that cold night, the drugs concealed all the turmoil inside me.

All of the calls were routine with brief small chat, time in the bed, mini-blowjob with a condom on, and sex to finish off the call. Generally, the men didn't want to kiss, but some tried, and I was not interested. Keeping my face away from theirs was a high priority. For me, kissing was the one thing I saved in my heart as an intimate gesture. It was an opportunity to look into someone's eyes and share the moment, feel their presence, and offer yours. Detaching from the moment with my clients meant I could not be present, and kissing was therefore forfeited.

Once I had a guy who asked if I would do anal, something I had only done a few times with guys of my choosing in my personal life and not something I had enjoyed. He offered me extra money, and I decided to give it a try. This particular client ran a wedding bonbonniere store in Toronto, and I'd seen him a few times already. I met him at the shop after hours, and we did the call right in the middle of the store on the floor beneath the tables of packaged candies, picture frames, and candles.

I got through the anal on that particular call but decided never to do it again; the pain of unwanted anal sex was not worth the extra money. Another guy wanted me to pee on him. It was something I had never done, but I knew my girl Jordy was a pro at it and laughed at what easy money it was to make, so I gave it a try. We spent the entire one-hour session in his bathroom, him laying naked in the tub and me squatting naked over him, trying to relax enough to golden shower his face. Like anal, this was not something I ever tried again. I managed to squeeze out a few drops but could not relax enough to offer the full experience a client looked for. Of course, once I was alone behind closed doors, it all came flying out of me. I had no specialities to offer, basic package only, which suited me just fine.

5

What Is Love?

While Jordy and I lived together at Martin and Carrie's, we met at the end of the night to get high. Jordy and I went on coke binges that sometimes lasted as little as one night, or they continued for days until we ran out of drugs and money. We had a serving platter on the bed she had stolen from the kitchen. It rotated, and she spun a line of powder around to me after she cut them and had inhaled her own. Jordy was a caretaker. I needed her to love and care for me, and she was the only person in my life who I felt had my back. She rose to the occasion and always made sure I stayed safe and had everything I needed. Jordy loved the preparation of the drugs, and I loved being pampered, so our roles in getting high aligned perfectly. She took total control in buying, setting up, and keeping the party going.

Sometimes, we got into deep conversations, but usually, by the end of the bag, we felt frozen with fear. The fear of coming down was extremely painful both mentally and physically. We felt the fear of the feelings of worthlessness, emptiness, and recognition of the poor choices we made. Curling up together in our shared bed, we silently waited out the storm listening to CDs on her stereo. Favourites to ease the discomfort were moody albums from Portishead, The Cranberries, and Tracey Chapman. I waited to hear her breathing slow into a steady rhythm, knowing she was temporarily at peace, and I silently thanked the universe for easing her pain while I waited for sleep myself.

On nights when I was alone, I found comfort in having her belongings with me; I listened to our favourite songs alone as I waited for her to return. We shared everything—clothes, bras, and even underwear. We had a sisterly bond, one that drugs and our inner demons eventually broke.

When I wasn't with Jordy, I was usually with my best guy friend, Denny. We were terrible for each other, and he had a gigantic appetite for cocaine. He was a local dealer, and our relationship was toxic. I cannot for the life of me remember how we met. We were probably introduced as customer/dealer, hit it off, and then stuck together like glue. Denny truly cared about me, and I believe he gave me a lot of free coke for multiple reasons. One of which was that he didn't want to be alone. Who better to have at your side than a hot, sex addict who would party with you for days? He didn't like that I was prostituting, so the free drugs kept me away from it and eased his mind. He had developed strong feelings for me, but he knew I didn't want to get into a committed relationship. Settling for the crumbs I had to offer him, occasionally we had sex. More often, though, I let him go down on me and then turned him away for anything else. I gave him only enough to hold his interest but not enough to become too attached.

In 1997, I moved in with Phaedra. She lived above a nail salon on Yonge Street in the north end of Toronto. I had stayed there during party benders and eventually met Eric, who would steal me away from Martin and Carrie to become my new pimp. I didn't keep the fact that I escorted private, and he approached me already knowing what I was doing. He was 21, I was 17, and it started as a "let's hook up" kind of encounter. He was very curious about my profession and how it worked. I explained that an ad with a description of my services and appearance was posted to a specific newspaper. The ad also had a number to call the agency, and once the client booked the appointment, a driver provided by the agency took me to the call. I split the money with the agency. Eric was money-hungry, and this perked up his ears. "Why don't we work together?" he asked. "I can post your ads and drive you to and from the calls; we'll make a great team."

I fell head over heels for him the moment he locked his beautiful blue eyes on me.

Eric was Russian, tall and lean, with short brown hair that had a slight wave to it. His hair and nails were always perfectly manicured, and he had a smile that could melt ice. He looked like the type of guy you took home to meet Momma. On the surface, he could charm you and make you feel like the only girl in the world. Now, I see him as a master manipulator, someone who would break my heart harder than anyone ever had. With feelings of infatuation for my new friend, I took him up on his offer immediately, which meant I needed to move out of the condo in Scarborough.

Moving at this stage of my life was incredibly easy. All I had to do was grab my duffle bag, load it up with whatever clothes I hadn't lost along the way, and off I went. I still had a bedroom at my parents' house that I left things at. Sometimes, I rotated through what was coming with me after stopping in for a sleepover that gave me a place to do laundry and have one of my mom's great home-cooked meals.

I set myself up at Phaedra's apartment; she was happy to have the company, and she had a crush on Eric. He was great at getting his way with women of low self-worth. She had a futon in her one-bedroom apartment that would be my new bed. She smoked a lot of weed, and there was a constant flow of bodies, usually men, passing through her place. There were a few apartments there, and it seemed that most of the tenants liked to party, so it was a regular place to hook up to do drugs, hang out before heading to a party or club, or chill and smoke weed during the week.

When Eric and I were together, I felt on top of the world. He drove me where I needed to go, my calls, the mall, nail salon, even my parents' house occasionally. Our relationship was weird. It felt like he was my boyfriend because he controlled so much of my life. He told me he loved me, and I believed him. I worked when he was available, did drugs when he said it was ok, and I only hung out with people he approved of. He really started controlling my drug use when he began selling cocaine. Some nights, he gave me as much as I wanted, and others he told me I was doing too much and needed to take a break. He gave off the impression that he cared about me, but now I see that this was his way of gaining complete control. When he told me he loved me, he made me feel like we were a couple. It was rare that he wouldn't respond to me paging him, and on the occasions he didn't, most likely out with another girl, I forgave him the instant I saw his handsome face or heard his voice, which had me eating out of the palm of his hand.

Jordy and I were still in touch and partying together as often as we could. I imagine she felt a bit slighted when I left to be with Eric. Even though she and I weren't a couple, we were connected on a soul-deep level that made me feel like we were bonded for eternity. With our addictions raging, I jumped at the opportunity to join one of her calls right down the street from the Yonge Street apartment. This was by far the craziest appointment I ever had. She had already been there all night, and her customer wanted her to spend the day. They were high, and she wanted to stay to continue earning easy money, but he was getting really weird and she needed back up.

She came to pick me up in a cab, and we headed to the bank with his card to withdraw money for our services and more cocaine. When we got back to his apartment, he paced around frantically, waiting for both the drugs and his company. My friend Denny met us in the lobby of the building to restock, and I could tell he was worried and didn't want me to stay. That wasn't an option, though. We grabbed the drugs and headed upstairs to the party. Line after line went up our noses. The client was a real freak, and he asked us to tie him up. We obliged because the pacing and frantic behaviour really tripped us out. Up to that point, I hadn't even touched him; he only wanted people to get high with.

Jordy had one of the best smiles I've ever seen, and as she grabbed neckties to start fastening him to his chair, I knew she was up to something. As he sat there naked and tied to a chair, she laughed at him and began to get dressed, encouraging me to do the same. I threw my clothes on as quickly as I could, and she collected all of the drugs and money. *We are going to rob him and leave him tied to the chair?* Yes, that's exactly what we did, running out of the penthouse condo with him yelling wildly after us. We laughed, both scared and excited, as we rushed onto the elevator and made our way down. When we got to the parking lot, we stopped for a moment to grasp what we planned to do next. We were suddenly shocked to see the guy come exploding out of the main entrance, naked, and yelling at us to come back. Terrified, we ran away and never looked back.

I had called Eric to pick us up and drive us to the Yonge Street apartment.

It took us hours to settle down. I'd never had a paranoia trip that bad. Every minute, we looked out the peephole expecting to see his wild face there ready to kill us. Every little sound made us jump as we tried to sit as silently as possible so no one would know we were there consuming every last piece of dust in the coke bag. The comedown was a hard one, but then they always were.

Eric had a friend he wanted to introduce Jordy to, saying he would be great to manage her escorting. They met and hit it off, so now Jordy and I grew closer again. She posted her new ads with her new friend, and the old agency found out and went crazy. She had to pull a quick move-out from their condo with a friend she took with her to intimidate them into releasing her belongings. Now, Jordy needed a place to stay, so the two pimps put us up together in a motel called The Emerald Isle.

We planned to do in-call services there all weekend long, but the only thing we serviced was our noses full of cocaine. We went on a crazy bender, and it fuelled one of our biggest fights ever. Stuck in that room together for days, high out of our minds, our friendship edged to the brink of destruction. She'd had enough of my shit, and I'd had enough of hers. After she left, I sat on the bed and sobbed uncontrollably. I cried because of how unmanageable my life had become, how I had lost my only friend, and how I was in love with someone I knew didn't love me back.

Eric came to my rescue as he always did, and we decided to rent a basement apartment together. I was so excited at the idea of moving in with him and thought that maybe my dreams of us being together forever were going to come true. We went to view the apartment together, fronting as an average couple. We told them I was in school and worked part-time and that he was the manager of a gas station, which was true. He had many different avenues of income, and I would imagine he is successful today based on his love for money.

Eric brought a few furnishings from his parents' basement at home: a love seat chair and TV to go with the existing kitchen table with two chairs. He also brought an old mattress with some blankets, and I brought my bag of clothes. It was nice to have my own space finally and not be at the mercy of other people. When we acquired the apartment, I had no idea how much it would be my own place. Eric never spent a single night there. He came over every day after work and on his days off, but he never stayed; he always went home to his parents' house to sleep. This kept me on my toes and was another part of his masterful manipulation. It made me miss him and wait like a little puppy dog for his return; I had turned into his puppet. I followed his instructions exactly, and he made sure I had everything I needed. He brought me food and spent just enough time with me to keep me satisfied, he continued to drive me anywhere I needed to go, and he took half of the money I made escorting. I really liked being irresponsible; I was more than happy to give him complete control. The fewer decisions I had to make about my life, the less I had to worry about what was going to happen to me. I believed he loved me, but I had never had a good example of what love was. Often left wondering if the control and manipulation were normal in a relationship but figured it must be as my feelings for him were so strong.

One weekend, Eric left me alone at the apartment. Before he took off, I started feeling unwell and saw his concern for me. My stomach ached, and I had a slight fever. He promised he would come back in the evening after he attended a party his parents were hosting. I busied myself around the tiny apartment, cleaning obsessively as I often did to pass the time: dusting, washing up the dishes, and I even cleaned the bathroom while trying to ignore the growing pain in my stomach. After taking a few Tylenol, I lay down on my pathetic mattress to sleep it off. This was not to be slept off.

The pain increased, and I curled up in the fetal position, trying to soothe myself in the darkness of the windowless bedroom.

My senses were on high alert: I could smell the dampness of the room, and it made me nauseous. I decided to get up and run a hot bath to help ease my pains, and I lay in the tub for a long while. When the water started to turn lukewarm, I began to pick myself up to exit the tub, but I could barely stand. I grabbed a towel, sat on the bathmat, and started to cry. My head started to boil, and I realized I had a high fever. I got to the toilet and vomited. Something was seriously wrong, but I had no clue what kind of flu it was. I had never had this type of pain before. I called Eric, and when he realized this was serious, he hurried over to bring me to the hospital. He dropped me off at the front like a taxi would have and told me to call him as soon as I was done. He winked and blew me a kiss, and I forgave him instantly for not being there for me.

I entered emergency at Humber River Hospital alone. My fever was extremely high, and I moaned in extreme discomfort, tears and all. They took me in quickly, assuming it was my appendix. An x-ray revealed I had something lodged deep inside my vagina. The doctor said he needed to perform a pap test to try to fish out whatever was stuck. I could barely believe it when he pulled out a condom; I was mortified. He wondered how I didn't know there was a condom left behind and felt as though my boyfriend should have said something. I pretended I was in shock that my boyfriend didn't tell me. In reality, it could have been from any of the multiple encounters I'd had that week. They ran a battery of tests for STDs and pregnancy, all coming back negative. Then, I was put on antibiotics, and they sent me on my way. I took a taxi home and crawled into my pathetic bed once again and cried myself to sleep, feeling so alone, completely hopeless, and desperate to find my way in the world. Drugs and prostitution held me hostage, and Eric had me exactly where he wanted me, like a puppet waiting for a cue on how to behave, who to be friends with, and where and when I partied.

Denny and I were still friends, and he was also friendly with Eric. I did have restrictions on how much time I was allowed to spend with Denny, but if Eric was busy and didn't have time to monitor me, he left me with Denny as my babysitter. Usually, he returned to pick me up, and he'd be disappointed with how high and dishevelled I was. He gave me a stern look of disapproval, made me feel guilty, but he always smiled when I apologized and promised not to get out of hand again. We both knew this was a lie, but we accepted this as truth to maintain our roles.

For my eighteenth birthday, Eric dropped me off at my parents' house to have dinner with them. My mom always asked me what I wanted, and I either chose lasagna or home-made macaroni with cheese and ham. My mother was an amazing cook and baker; she instilled these skills in me to use at a later date. My parents thought I worked at a bedding store. One day while I was out driving somewhere with Eric, I was on the phone with my mom, and she asked how I was and if I had a job. I saw the sign to Beddington's on Yonge Street and said, "Yes, I do have a job—at Beddington's." She gobbled up my bullshit, wanting to believe it was true.

They never asked to meet Eric, and Eric never asked to meet my parents. They had met so many of my fucked-up friends and boyfriends along the way, and I'm sure they were more than content with me not bringing this one home. They only asked if I was happy and that everything was ok. I assured them everything was great and that I was very happy. On this birthday, after having a homemade birthday cake, I opened my present.

I still have it to this day and am wearing it now: a white gold necklace with a pendant of a cursive capital D with tiny diamonds encrusting it. It was my favourite piece of jewellery, and I wore it every day. Recently, I went over my fears with my husband about writing my story and sharing my struggles publicly, questioning if I had made the right decision. He said I needed a North Star, something I can look at to ground me and remind me of the importance of my work. I had seen the necklace in my drawer a few weeks prior while searching for something and immediately thought of it. This was a period in my life I had been desperately trying to hide and forget, but it was such a big part of my life story that it was never going to disappear. The necklace was the only physical item I still owned from that time in my life. Putting it on and looking in the mirror, I decided that whenever I felt these fears and doubts, I could reach for the pendant. It would remind me that my story was not one to be erased. This was going to be a story of resilience that needed to be shared. I would turn my pain into purpose.

Later that evening, I got into Eric's car with my presents and a smile on my face. He looked at me with sadness in his eyes and said, "Dee, why are you escorting? You have a family that cares about you, you're beautiful, and so much better than what you are living." I smiled at him and turned to look silently out the window; I didn't have an answer. All I knew was that I felt like I was drowning in a big, scary world. I was confused about love, life, and what I was going to do with myself. I just wanted to get high so I didn't have to think about it all.

6

The Breakup

Eric and I carried on for a few more months of outcalls, and our pretend relationship. I had a regular who I saw weekly; he had taken a strong liking to me. Andrew was in his fifties and desperately hanging onto his youth. He loved having me over and always wanted to chat; eventually, we became friends, though he saw it as something more. It was nice to have regulars, as this provided a steadier income. The business would ebb and flow, busy at times and completely dry at others.

One sunny afternoon, Eric and I drove south on Yonge Street; he had just picked me up at my mother's house. We got into a bit of an argument, and he scolded me. I could see him grasping for control over me, but it was slipping from his grasp. The look on his face before he smacked me in the back of the head I will never forget; it was a look of desperation. I had never seen him afraid before; something was changing. The smack to the back of the head was a shock; he had never hit me before, other than the odd aggressive grab to my face when speaking to me to drive a point home. The next thing I knew, I flew into the front windshield. During our argument, Eric had rear-ended the car ahead of us, and I wasn't wearing my seatbelt. I sat back in my seat and looked over to him and saw deep concern in his eyes. My head was bleeding, and I started to cry. He scrambled to make sure I was ok, and I was. We had reached a new level of dysfunction in our relationship. Funny enough, the accident happened right in front of a walk-in clinic. The doctor came running out to check on me and rushed me into his office. After a thorough check-up, I was fine, the cut was superficial, and I didn't need stitches. The doctor eyed Eric suspiciously, asked him to drive more carefully, and off we went.

A few weeks after this incident, while I was visiting my parents for a few days, Eric called and told me he was breaking things off with me. He wanted me to move on to better things and told me we would never see each other again. I was devastated. He was my whole world; I was planning a life with him. He hung up the phone, and I immediately called him back to no answer. I called again and again, and he wouldn't pick up. I dropped to my knees and screamed out the hollow pain I felt in my stomach. My world had collapsed, and I didn't know how to cope. I called Denny and told him I needed to see him right away. The only way I knew how to cope was by drowning out my feelings of low self-worth with massive amounts of drugs. Denny was always there for me anytime I called. He could have been with the hottest girl on earth, but I was his kryptonite. He came to me in a heartbeat to save the day. Of course, we got high for days, cocaine in lines, cocaine in cigarettes, and cocaine in joints. We holed up at a sleazy motel in the north end of Richmond Hill called The Night's Inn.

When the party supplies ran out, I got down on my hands and knees to crawl around on the disgusting bathroom floor, as I had on many occasions, looking to find the tiny rocks of cocaine I never saw fall but prayed they had. There are plenty of little white rocks on dirty bathroom floors, by the way. I would taste test them all, mostly plaster and god knows what else. You are at a very low point in your life when you do the bathroom floor crawl. I was desperate, dishevelled, and damaged. We stayed at The Inn until 10 a.m., waiting for Denny's mom to leave for work so we would have the house to ourselves. Denny and I were on day five of a serious bender. We each ate a half-quarter of mushrooms and smoked a huge joint.

We were out of blow and decided we needed to come down and get some sleep. Not sure why we thought mushrooms were going to be our saviour, but we were just desperate not to feel the earthquake of a comedown that was hitting us *hard*. We lay in his bed and decided to fuck, hoping an orgasm would help. I noticed it had helped him when I heard him talking Portuguese and saying mama over and over again in a real stupor of sleep. *Asshole.* Suffering and thinking death would be better than mourning the loss of my child named cocaine, I moved into the fetal position and tried to console my broken self.

Suddenly, I heard yelling downstairs. Men's voices shouted, "Denny, Denny! Where are you? I know you're here!"

I was terrified. "Denny, wake up! There is someone here! Denny!" He mumbled away in Portuguese as I shook him awake. He finally came to, looking incredibly confused and still fucked up. As he started to realize there were people in his house looking for him, he became more alert and jumped out of bed and into a pair of track pants. He closed the bedroom door behind him as he headed downstairs. I heard the voices talking to him. They were looking for drugs, and when they realized how much of a mess Denny was, they poked fun at him. Denny spoke half-English/half-Portuguese and still said mama every once in a while.

"Denny, you're fucked, buddy. What the fuck is wrong with you?" they said. I recognized that voice … it was Matt. We had met at Phaedra's awhile back; his was not a voice you would ever forget, or face for that matter. Matt was 6'4" with ice blue piercing eyes and long blonde hair pulled back into a ponytail. He was striking; you couldn't miss him in a crowd. He was cocky, and we chatted for a bit, but I was Eric's girl at the time, so neither of us pursued anything.

"Where is Deirdre?" I heard him say. "I know she's here— where is she?"

Shit. Fuck. This can't be happening. I had just come down from one of the biggest benders of all time, and I had to deal with this shit. *No one can see me like this: I haven't slept in five days.* Full of anxiety from my comedown, fear and adrenaline now joined the party. I jumped into Denny's closet and closed the door.

As they came up the stairs, I heard, "*Bro,* she's not here. I was sleeping. You need to get out of here. My mom is on her way home." Denny pled with him as they ascended the staircase. I held my breath and made myself as small as possible in the dark closet. The door opened. "No one is here. Come on, man, you need to go," Denny pleaded again.

"Matt, let's get out of here!" his friend yelled from the bottom of the stairs. The footsteps moved away from the bedroom, and I heard them make their way downstairs. Phew! That was close. *What the heck does he want with me?* I thought. Maybe he heard that Eric and I had parted ways and wanted to hook up.

Denny returned, looking utterly defeated. We barely spoke at that point; our brains short-circuited, our words scrambled, and we couldn't string together a sentence. We lay down and passed out from all the excitement.

We woke up a few hours later to Denny's mom yelling in Portuguese. She was going on and on, sounding very upset. Denny assured me that was normal for her; she communicated loudly. He headed downstairs to say hello and got us some food. I already knew I wasn't supposed to be there, and he expected me to stay quiet. I didn't plan on leaving and knew it was going to be a long evening of hiding out in his room.

We had not slept off our binge enough, and I struggled to function. As we had our snack and rested, we listened to all the sounds of his busy house now that his dad and sister also came home. I'd been in this situation more times than I can remember: hiding in someone's house or having someone hide in mine. Later in the evening, we heard his mom's footsteps coming toward the door, and I quietly slipped back into the closet. She checked up on him because she thought it was suspicious that he'd been in his room all evening. Finally, the house quieted, and we settled into bed. He smiled at me, and his adoration for me showed in his eyes. I always thought Denny was so sweet but looked at him as more of a brother than a lover. He always made me feel safe with him, and we slipped into a sleep that would let us recover from our binge.

I needed a permanent place to live. Making a deal with my parents that I would go to night school to pick up a few credits seemed like a good option. I wasn't partying as much, and I was making an effort to do better. I was still seeing my regular Andrew who would give me some extra cash; picking me up occasionally to spend an afternoon together. He took me shopping and bought me expensive gifts, mostly clothes, shoes, and purses. The cash he gave me was just enough to get me by without having to find a job or go back to prostitution. He even bought me a dog one day while we were shopping at Yorkdale one afternoon.

When I walked in, I saw the most beautiful, sad-looking puppy. He had red hair and big baby blue eyes. A Dogue de

Bordeaux—a French Mastiff that would grow into a 140-pound drooling beast. I had to have him. We took him out of his crate and cuddled him; my heart sang. I had been so lonely and was desperately looking for love. This was my most expensive gift yet, costing $3,000. We picked out everything I needed, and I took that dog home to my parents' house. It's a good thing my dad loves dogs, but that's not to say they were impressed. In no way were they happy to be hosting a puppy. They did let him stay, though, and I took care of him like he was my baby. I trained him quickly to use the bathroom outdoors, even setting my alarm twice through the night to get up with him and head outside for his pee. I named him Fitzroy, and he was my companion for seven years until he suddenly passed away in his sleep.

I had my dog, but I still longed for human connection. One weekend, I was out partying with Denny, and we ran into Matt, the tall, icy blue-eyed guy who stormed through Denny's house weeks before. He swung by to pick up drugs from Denny, who was selling coke, weed, and heroin. His eyes locked on me right away, and we talked for a while. We exchanged numbers and off he went with his friends. I was intrigued by him. He was loud, confident, and intimidating. I needed to feel safe and protected, so this was very attractive to me. He called me that same weekend and asked to meet up. He was heading to the Comfort Zone and asked me to meet him there. (Comfort Zone was an after-hours club in Toronto where drug addicts spent their daytime hours in a dark, dirty dungeon.)

They played good music, and I wanted to see him. I had spent the night at my friend Kerry's—yes, the ex-girlfriend: she didn't touch hard drugs and was helping me through the horrible come down from the night before. When we woke, I spoke with Matt and then asked her if she wanted to go. She was in! *Yes!* Kerry had a car, making it easy to get down there. We got all done up and headed downtown to dance and have fun. I hung out with Matt, and everything was great. We stayed all day until the club shut down. When we went outside, I saw Matt walking away from the club with two girls. My heart sank. He wasn't interested in me. We drove back up to Richmond Hill, and I thought, *Fuck him! He's missing out.*

Night school didn't last long; I went for a month or so, but I couldn't hack it. Being in class, I felt trapped. If anyone forced me to do anything, my instinct was always to fight back. I was seeing someone casually for sex, and he picked me up after class or brought me to school if we'd hooked up earlier. Sex with him was amazing, but I don't remember his name. I don't remember a lot of their names, and there were many.

Without attending school, I needed to get a job, or my parents would threaten to kick me out. I found a telemarketing gig in the mall near my house. Perfect. Matt also connected with me again, and I decided to give it another chance. I was attracted to him, so why not?

Another chance turned into a few months of dating, partying, and using lots of drugs. Cleaning myself up was off the table as we went full force stuffing blow up our noses and smoking heroin to bring us back down. It was a dance, the coke and the heroin weaving together. I didn't really like heroin; I preferred to be full of the cocaine confidence. It made me feel invincible until the hard comedown, and that's when I learned to appreciate its dance partner. Matt and I started smoking crack together as well. I had already tried it a few times in the past, but we were going all the way. We had sex constantly, becoming as addicted to each other as we were the drugs.

Matt worked with me at the call centre for a brief period. I have no idea how either of us held down that job. We had a short evening shift, 4 p.m.–8 p.m.; I think that's the only reason we were able to manage it.

Shit hit the fan that summer when I realized I was pregnant. We weren't using any protection, and I was shocked, scared, and unsure of what to do. Both of us used massive amounts of drugs again; I barely worked, had no education, and really had only started dating this guy. *Did I want to settle down with him? Could I trust him? How would we support ourselves?* So many questions swirled around in my head.

When I told my mom I was pregnant, she was angry and very concerned. She had been a single mother herself at the age of nineteen and didn't want me to face the same struggles. She said she supported whatever decision I made, but I felt she was leaning toward the abortion side of the equation.

Matt also told his mother, Maya. His family was Catholic, and abortion was not on the table for them at all. Ultimately, the decision was mine to make, and I decided to have an abortion. Matt threatened that if I went that route, he would break up with me. He was true to his word.

The walk-in clinic I had gone to for the pregnancy test gave me all of the information on the abortion clinic, and I booked myself an appointment.

Walking into that clinic felt so strange. Looking at the other girls, knowing they were about to embark on the same path, seemed like such an intrusion. My heart ached for them and myself, but I knew this was the right decision for me. They had me remove my clothes and put on a hospital gown after a brief interview where the nurse asked me at least four times if I was sure that this was what I wanted to do. My answer was unwavering: yes, I was having an abortion. They gave me a sedative to help me relax. When it was my turn, I walked into the room and lay down on the table, feet in stirrups, legs spread, nerves on high alert. *Is this going to be painful? How long will it take? What if I regret it?* I closed my eyes and removed myself from my body, a skill acquired from the sex trade. The doctor said, "Just relax. Imagine you're only here for a pap test." It was over quickly, a bit painful but not what I had imagined. They gave me a giant maxi pad to put in my underwear and took me to the recovery room.

The following days, I bled heavily, more than a period, and I felt a little weepy. The cramps were ferocious, and I used Advil to help manage the pain.

Going into the call center was difficult because Matt still worked there. He was not a nice person if you were on his bad side and had no problem calling me a bitch as I passed by him. I didn't let him intimidate me and kept on with my business. I made a few new friends there and even started dating one of my co-workers as a distraction. Eventually, Matt quit, and I breathed easier when going to work.

7

Prison Sentence

By the end of summer 1998, Matt had reached out to me, wanting to reconcile. The boyfriend I had was on the tame side, and while it was fun shocking him with how adventurous I was, it wasn't enough to keep me hooked. Matt's specialty was excitement and adventure. He would be my kryptonite. We immediately returned to heavy drug use, going to clubs and having endless amounts of sex. It wasn't long before I quit my call center job and became a full-time druggie once again. My parents weren't having it, so I moved in with Matt and his mother.

His dad had been out of the picture since he was a little boy. He had moved here with his mom and aunt, Maya's twin, from Poland when he was ten. They lived in a housing project, but this one was clean with no bugs. Fitzroy came along with me; thankfully, Matt took him on as his own, and Maya loved him too. I don't know how his mother put up with us coming and going as we pleased. We stayed up all night, and we smoked cigarettes, weed, crack, and heroin in the apartment.

They fought constantly in Polish, and he didn't back down. While his mother was a tough cookie, he eventually won her over either with charm or intimidation. When one wasn't working, he tried the next until he wore her down.

Matt and I fought a lot too. I can't even remember why, but the moodiness of two drug addicts was enough to ignite tempers. One night after going out partying, we got a ride home from the friends we had gone out with. Lina, a friend from a few years back, got out of the car to hug me, and we kissed passionately. She was a fantastic kisser and had beautiful, soft lips. As we pulled away from each other, Matt comes in and punches me in the stomach. I doubled over and fell back to the ground.

I heard a commotion, and a group of guys ran at him. Someone hit him over the back of the head with a crowbar, and he dropped to the ground. They had been hanging out across the street and saw him assault me. "Get out of here! I've called the police," someone yelled from a balcony up above. *Shit.* My friends sped off in the car, and Matt and I hurried in to take the elevator upstairs. It wasn't long before the police were at our door. I assured them I was fine and that he had never hit me. I told them we had just been arguing when these guys came up and attacked him.

It seemed like every weekend was full of drama; we fought like cats and dogs. One night, I had packed all of my stuff into two bags and walked along Finch Avenue with Fitzroy to the closest gas station where I sat down to figure out what to do next. He was so verbally abusive; I knew that staying was wrong, but I didn't have the strength or support to leave. I knew my parents didn't want me at home, and I didn't want to be under their roof again either. Matt pulled up in his souped-up Honda Civic, and in his cocky, no-nonsense way told me to "get the fuck in the car." So, I did. I truly felt like I wasn't going to find better, and I was so scared to be on my own. Unfortunately, I was used to being someone's property, a lesson I had falsely learned so long ago—men had power over women, and we were their objects. I needed intervention on every level: someone to lead me to a new path. It would be years before my healing process would begin.

I decided to get a job and had a resume made to hand out around Fairview Mall. A clothing store responded, and I went in for an interview. I got the job! I was excited to get out on my own and start making a little bit of my own money. Not surprisingly, I only made it to two shifts. The first shift, I went in sober and managed okay. The second shift, I went in after a night of no sleep and high on heroin; I left during my break and never returned. I was so full of insecurities, making it impossible for me to get my shit together for even a few hours. Holding down a job and doing drugs full time was not an easy task. Matt managed to maintain his job okay, though; he was a high-functioning addict and could shut the party down to go to work and get shit done. He did deliveries, and that meant Fitzroy and I could join him; we waited in the car while he completed the delivery part, mostly envelopes and small packages.

Matt had extreme road rage, and he got into verbal fights with drivers constantly. He always tailgated, cut people off, blasted his horn, and acted as rude as anyone could be. I once saw him pull over, and someone drove their truck into the open driver side door. (I'm not sure how it didn't come off!) The door was still usable, but we drove on to chase them. He also held a baseball bat out the window as a threat, tapped cars with his car, and swore and yelled and made an absolute ass out of himself so many times. It was exhausting, and when he started raging, there was no bringing him down. I just got quiet, which I was very good at, and tried to disappear inside myself, hoping he wouldn't get us killed.

In November, I found out I was pregnant again. I'd missed my period for a few months but ignored it, thinking it was because of all of the heavy drug use, poor diet, and stress. No, against all of these odds, we had created a baby. I immediately thought this was meant to be. A baby was trying hard to come into this world through me, and I would honour that. I asked the nurse who gave me the news if the baby would be okay and explained to them I had been using a lot of drugs, drinking alcohol, and smoking. The nurse said that if I quit everything that day, the odds were in favour of having a completely healthy, beautiful baby. So, that's what I did; I quit everything cold turkey, dedicating my body to that baby. Thankfully, I realized I needed to make a lot of changes quickly. I was already two and a half months pregnant and had absolutely nothing going for me. Needing stability, I asked my parents if I could move back home if I got a full-time job. They agreed, and I followed through.

I got a job at Grand and Toy, an office supplies company in Hillcrest Mall, which was where the call centre was. It was only a ten-minute walk away, and I had a Monday–Friday shift from 9 to 4. It was perfect. I saved every penny I made aside from the $500 per month my parents charged me for room and board. Matt started snow removal in the winter and gave me part of his pay to stash away. He said he was getting sober as well and attended a day treatment program, but I knew he was slipping but had no proof. I remained focused on myself, worked, rested, saved, and waited. I still hadn't told my mother that the change in my life was because I was pregnant.

One night, Mactt was over, and he wanted to smoke a joint. I said no: if I couldn't, then he couldn't. Well, he was not someone who took demands or rules well. He was livid that I was trying to control him. Wanting to avoid the fight, I left the basement and joined my mother in the sunroom at the back of the house. She was watching her evening program and enjoying a cup of tea. Matt walked in, sat down, and said, "Hey, Deirdre, why don't you tell your mother that your fuckin' pregnant?" with a giant smirk on his face. Forever an asshole. My mother was not impressed; she glared at me and asked if it was true.

"Yes, it is, and I'm keeping the baby."

She said, "Don't let your father find out. Let's get through Christmas, and then we will tell him."

It turned out my oldest brother was buying a house and would be moving out of his apartment two weeks before the baby was due. He offered to sublease the place to me, which meant I got to keep the low monthly rental rate. He had been living there for ten years, and the law in Ontario was you could only increment a small percentage every year. This meant I would get a huge two-bedroom apartment for less than the average cost of a one-bedroom apartment. No dogs were allowed, but he assured me they couldn't evict me; it was more of a deterrent. Things were looking up. I had money saved, an apartment lined up, and I was healthy again. Matt's mom decided that since we would be moving in together, she would go live with her twin sister. She gave us her couches, TV, and some dishes.

I bought everything else we needed at Ikea, a futon bed, dressers, and the extra kitchen supplies. My mom had a kitchen table in storage I had eaten at as a baby, and Maya gave us chairs to go with it. My biggest problem was Matt. His behaviour was getting worse: vile language, not taking my calls, slowly giving me less money. I knew he was back on drugs. I called him on it and told him I wouldn't speak to him until he cleaned himself up. One night when I was eight months pregnant, he wouldn't answer the phone, and I imagined he was out with another girl. I never got proof, but his mother confirmed he never came home that night.

That last month of my pregnancy, we still fought, and I didn't trust him. I wouldn't take his calls; I was so tired of his shit.

While I was in the front yard with Fitzroy enjoying the beautiful spring day, his car drove by the house. He passed by, but I knew he would come back. Pulling up, he asked me to get in. "Let's talk," he said. I decided to go along with it to see what he had to say. He wanted a fight; we argued immediately, and he started up the car and raced around the neighbourhood. Pulling over at one point, he pulled out a pop can and took a few hits of crack, right there in the car with me eight months pregnant.

I started to panic as I could tell he was out of his mind. Scrambling, I tried to open the door to get out, but he started driving again, so I shut the door quickly. He drove over curbs and onto people's front lawns; he also bluffed that he would drive into things, like mailboxes and lampposts. He wanted to scare me to the core, and he succeeded. I couldn't understand how someone who said they loved me could behave that way. After an hour of this torture, he finally dropped me off at home. I was crushed.

Days later, I got a call from him saying he had been arrested for assaulting a police officer who had pulled him over. I wasn't surprised. When they ran his fingerprints, he matched a home invasion that had happened the year prior, and they booked him on that. Apparently, when we were broken-up for that month or so, he had committed the crime. I learned that he'd intended to break into my friend Jordy's apartment, looking for someone who owed him money for a large amount of crystal meth. Except he'd entered the wrong apartment and ended up in the bedroom of a terrified couple who had no idea what was happening. Matt touched a CD and left a fingerprint. He also found Jordy's apartment next door and ransacked that as well.

Matt's lawyer suggested he take anger management classes and go back to a drug treatment program to show the courts he was seeking help for his troubles. We hoped it would result in a reduced sentence. A dark cloud hung over our heads from that day forward. His sentencing would be a few months after our baby was born. At least he wouldn't miss that, and with good programming, we were hopeful the court would be lenient on him.

On May 1st, 1999, we moved into our apartment. My mom decorated and painted the baby's room. We did a neutral teddy bear theme because we wanted to keep the gender a surprise. I was in major nesting mode, keeping the two-bedroom apartment spotless, cooking, and baking. Excitement was building for my little one to arrive. Matt was doing well with his programs, and things looked hopeful. Knowing his sentencing was coming up drew him in closer to me. He knew he needed support and wasn't going to screw things up again. On May 12th, I decided I was going to bake as many cinnamon loaves as I could and freeze them so we would have lots while I was busy with the new baby. When I finished my baking, I still had a lot of energy, so we went out to enjoy the beautiful spring evening and took Fitzroy for a long walk.

We came home late in the evening around 9 p.m. and started winding down for the night. At 11 p.m., the first contraction hit, and they started coming hard. "I'm having contractions, but I think I can go to sleep." I told Matt. I really did not want to go into labour; I was terrified. I lay down to try to sleep, but I jumped back up as soon as the next one hit, realizing there would be no sleeping through it. Matt called my mom as we had planned, and she made the thirty-minute drive from Richmond Hill to the north end of Toronto to pick us up and head back to Mackenzie Hospital in Richmond Hill. At 5:56 a.m., we had a baby girl, Monika. I spent the day and the next night in the hospital with that precious little babe; breastfeeding came naturally, and even though I had never cared for a baby in my life, I knew what to do and wasn't nervous. Of course, Matt headed out to the bar with his friends to celebrate. I didn't care, though. I had my baby girl.

The first few days at home were rough. Matt invited his friends over to celebrate, and they drank on the balcony. The second night, my bedroom window was open, and I heard them going on and on. Then, I heard him tell his friend to pee off the balcony, and I went out there and lost my shit. His friend surely thought I was crazy. Looking back, I definitely had some postpartum depression, but I didn't know anything about it at the time and didn't get help.

Otherwise, I adjusted easily to motherhood; it all came very natural to me. I breastfed and cuddled her all day long. I didn't miss my friends or the partying. Monika was my new addiction. I wanted to shower her with all of the love I felt had been missing from my life. Tending to her every need, I felt a great sense of fulfillment through caring for her. She was a very good baby, rarely crying for needs that could not be met. I viewed her as my precious princess and felt blessed that she had been born healthy.

When Monika was three months old, it was time for her father's court appearance. We went in hopeful. He had made a lot of improvements on himself to help his plea for less time. Matt had attended a day drug treatment program for the last few months, taken anger management, and was going to therapy. There was no mercy; they gave him six years, the maximum penalty for this crime. I was devastated. I thought, *How the heck am I supposed to do this on my own? Where is he going to go? What am I going to do?* They took him into custody right then and there. His mom, aunt, and I drove home in tears. They were quick to assure me that everything would be okay and that they were going to help me 100%.

I got back to my apartment and called my mom to tell her the news. She urged me to leave him. "Don't wait," she said. "Move on while you have the chance." I couldn't. Knowing he would be in there, scared and alone, I couldn't leave. He had my heart locked up in that prison with him. I would be loyal. I would wait. When he got out, we would continue. Matt called me every day, and we wrote letters back and forth. He started his sentence in a maximum-security prison in Kingston, Ontario. Knowing he was only allowed out of his cell for one hour each day was concerning. It killed me to picture him locked up in a tiny cell for twenty-three hours every day. His mom, Monika, and I would drive to Kingston, three hours each way, every weekend to visit.

Pulling up to the prison for the first time was a real eye-opener. The tall fences were doubled and had barbed wire at the top. Guards carrying guns were posted in towers, and we had to enter through many heavy steel doors that moved and locked with authority. In this prison, they assessed you to see where you belonged: maximum, medium, or minimum security. After a few months of good behaviour and positive feedback from counselling, Matt was sent to a minimum-security prison. This meant he would have free range of the property for most of the day and would be living in a dorm-style environment. He would order and cook his food, trade the orange jumpsuit for his own clothing, and our visits would be in the same room—no more glass and talking through the phone. We would be able to hug, hold hands, and he was going to be able to hold Monika.

8

Criminal University

Matt was now in a minimum-security prison in Gravenhurst, Ontario. It was a drastic change from the environment in Kingston. No big fences, no guards with guns, no heavy steel doors separating us from the prisoners. Instead, we pulled up to a small one-level building on our first visit. We walked through the front entrance into a cafeteria-style lounge full of tables and chairs. At one end was a front desk where we would check in. We were to show our ID, and they would search through our bags: Monika's diaper bag, our purses, and the picnic lunch bag. The guards wore plain clothes. Everything was so much more relaxed here, though the nerves of being inside a prison never entirely went away.

After ten minutes, Matt finally arrived at the visiting centre. He was dressed in his own clothes and had a huge smile and hug for us. I was so happy to have some physical contact finally and that he would be able to hold Monika, who was now six months old. The visits were for two to three hours, and we were even allowed outside. The visiting yard had a huge grassy area surrounded by forest. We enjoyed a huge lunch prepared by his aunt and hung out, keeping up a conversation easily.

We went to visit him every weekend, without fail, for over a year. Holidays were always a bit sad, and leaving was always hard. He had made some friends there and started working out. We were also unknowingly being schooled at Criminal University.

It began with a tattoo. He needed some parts to create the makeshift tattoo machine, and he needed ink. On one of our visits a month or so after he arrived, he asked me to smuggle these items in. At this point in my life, I had straightened myself out, but I thought ink and a few parts for a tattoo machine seemed pretty harmless. I decided to do it. Matt's friend on the outside met with me and gave me the items. Part one was super easy. Now for Part Two—getting it past the guards. I inserted the items into the diapers in the diaper bag I had brought for Monika. It was winter and Matt had a huge feather-filled jacket he would cut the liner in and put the items inside the coat. I was nervous, but nothing too upsetting, as the items I was bringing in weren't illegal. They just weren't allowed beyond the visitors' area of the prison.

The prisoners did get a quick pat-down on their way back into their area by an officer after the visits were over. They thoroughly searched pockets, shoes, and socks. I'm sure his walk back in was nerve-racking. I got my usual collect call from him later that night, and he let me know everything was fine; he passed through without suspicion. It was extremely relieving news, and he was excited to be getting his first tattoo. The first time I saw the beginning of it was in the spring, and we were laying outside of the visiting center on the grass. He rolled up his sleeve to show me his arm and chest. I was mortified and realized I had made a colossal mistake bringing him the contraband to get it started. It was only the outline; no detail had been done yet. It looked like a giant snake drawn by an amateur. I hated snakes—they totally creeped me out—and the head of this lizard was right on his chest. The body travelled over his shoulder and down his arm. Matt knew I was not impressed and assured me that when he was finished, it would look like a dragon that had been professionally done. I had my doubts. Thankfully, he proved me wrong, and the sloppy snake slowly turned into a magnificent dragon over the next few months.

Getting the tattoo contraband in so easily sparked Matt's interest in seeing what else he could sneak past the guards. One visit, he told me he wanted me to meet one of his friends on the outside to grab an ounce of weed. Then, he wanted me to package it in tiny balloons that he would swallow retrieve later once they'd passed through his system. I decided to go ahead with it. He would send me home some extra cash from this exchange, and I was really tight for money being on social assistance, so the opportunity seemed good. The next week, I met up with his friend to pick up the package. The weed was garbage, but it was free and better than not having anything.

Late that evening, after Monika was tucked in for the night, I started working on making the mini packages. I wrapped small amounts of the herbs in saran wrap, ran the flame from a lighter over it to seal it, and then wrapped it in a balloon, tying it tight. They were about the size of a thumbnail.

I made a big batch of chocolate pudding and put twenty balloons in it. I figured the dark colour would hide the balloons if, by chance, the guards opened the food, which they never did. The following day it was time to visit, and I was nervous. I packed the chocolate pudding in with the rest of the food and set off.

We went in to register, and as usual, the guards leafed through the bags and told us to go sit down and wait for Matt to come up. Holy shit, it worked! Phew, I was so relieved—the hardest part on my end was over, and it couldn't have been smoother. Matt came out with a huge smile and hugs. Then, he quickly asked, "Did you bring it?" I opened up our picnic lunch and showed him the big vat of pudding he was to consume to take his treasure over to the other side. He started to eat the dessert, and I cringed at the thought of him swallowing those little balloon packages, quickly removing the thought of the search party that would take place the next day to retrieve them. I couldn't imagine doing something like that! It takes a special kind of person to put themselves through that or maybe just a very desperate one. We finished our visit as usual, always one of the very last to go.

Again, I got my call later that evening, letting me know he was ok. The following day, Matt called back to let me know the packages had passed, and he had them in hand.

On our next visit, he had a new plan. He wanted to bring in larger quantities and coached me on how to prepare it. This time, the packages were going up his anus; I couldn't believe what I was hearing. "Are you serious?" I asked. He was.

We spent the rest of the visit going over the plan; he also wanted me to bring in alcohol, and we decided I would throw it into the garbage container in the women's bathroom. His friend was in charge of cleaning the visiting centre, and he would get it from there during his rounds. During visits, I met some of his friends when they also had family come to see them. It very quickly all became normalized. This was part of our lifestyle now—prison, crime, and meeting people to pick up packages. I didn't consider the depth of it or how much trouble I could get into until later down the road. It was all happening so gradually.

The following week, I had prepared the new packages like I was asked—long pellets around six inches in length and three fingers round. Again, in the evening, I prepared them the same way with saran wrap and fire-sealed them.

There were no balloons this time. I don't remember bringing lubrication, though I think it may have been a possibility. The liquor went in with the diapers, and I was very nervous going through security. This was the largest amount of contraband I had brought in: two large pellets of marijuana and a bottle of vodka. They barely checked my bags and had us take seats to wait. Matt came out wearing his big jacket. We all sat at the table together, and he put the diaper bag in his lap and transferred something from his jacket into the bag—$200 in one- and two-dollar coins. The prisoners only received change for their canteen, just enough to buy some treats if they were lucky enough to have family bring them money. They had been saving it up, and I was so happy to receive this money, as things had been really tight at home. I was living off of $1,200 per month through government assistance. He asked if I had the pellets, and I told him they were in the bag. He fished them out, put them in his coat, and headed to the bathroom. I winced, knowing he was about to insert those up his ass!

After he returned from the bathroom, he let me know everything worked out just fine. A sense of relief washed over me; he wasn't going to have to sneak it back in with the jacket and take a significant chance of getting us both busted. Now, it was my turn to head to the bathroom. I took Monika with me to change her diaper. Once she was all taken care of, I placed the liquor wrapped in diapers into the waste bin. I couldn't wait to get out of the prison that day. Getting back to the car, I felt the nerves finally settle and waited to hear from him that everything went ok on his side. He called that evening and let me know it had. His packages had arrived, and it was much easier to deal with in this new manor.

After being there for six months, he was allowed to have a conjugal visit. That meant that Monika and I would be able to visit for a weekend. They had two cabins on the property

for these types of visits. Of course, he had a list of contraband he wanted me to bring in. Alcohol, MDMA, steroids,
and hash were on the menu. I would go meet up with one
of his friends to pick up the product and pack plastic wrap
and lighters in my bags. He assured me he had a connection
with one of the guards who was going to make sure my bags
got passed through without inspection.

I was really excited about this visit; we'd have a whole
weekend together, hanging out and spending time with
Monika. My nerves were on high alert about bringing in
all of the contraband, but I trusted that he had everything
aligned in our favour and that I would be protected. My
mother-in-law drove Monika and I up and dropped us off
there. It was May, and the weather was feeling fresh and
rejuvenating. Seeing the first signs of spring budding up in
the dirt around the various garden beds on the property was
welcoming. I had been there so many times that I had a sense
of familiarity and belonging.

We unloaded my overnight bag along with a cooler of
pre-prepared food. Matt's favourites were all there: chicken
cutlets, mashed potatoes, green beans with bread crumbs,
and several desserts since he had a major sweet tooth. I had
also brought two bottles of wine, hash, steroids and MDMA
hidden in my carry-on. Upon arrival, we were asked to leave
the bags in the cabin and wait inside the main building for
Matt. I knew the bags were meant to be searched by guards,
and I silently prayed Matt's inside connection was true to
his word. Matt was called down, and they escorted us into
the cabin together. Our bags were sitting in on the floor and
looked as though they hadn't been touched. When the guards
left, I immediately went to check my belongings. Everything
was there! I couldn't believe we were getting away with it!
We unloaded the cooler, put the wine in the fridge, and I
showed Matt all of the goodies I had brought for him. He

was in heaven and quickly rolled up a hash joint and smoked it in the bathroom.

I hadn't used drugs since finding out I was pregnant and had no intention of starting. He was to enjoy that all to himself. I drank my wine and was very happy to indulge a little after Monika was put to bed for the night. We stayed up watching tv and hanging out. Funny, I don't remember having sex, though I know it happened. The next day, we ate, drank, watched tv, and he smoked the hash. Matt eventually turned one of the empty wine bottles into a hash bong by cracking a hole in the side bottom of the bottle. He put a piece of hash on a cigarette and stuck it into the hole. Then, he plugged the top of the bottle with his thumb until the entire thing filled up with thick, sweet smoke. Two large inhales, and he had it all sucked back, and I saw that he had thoroughly enjoyed his weekend.

On the second night, I started getting a little antsy, feeling a little suffocated by being in this small cabin, and I couldn't imagine having to live there on the property. We started getting on each other's nerves by the end of our visit. It was the most amount of time we had spent together in nine months, and I realized his shitty attitude was still very much alive. On the last morning, we woke up and started cleaning up the tiny cabin. I packed my bags with the empty wine bottles Matt had turned into hash bongs, lighters, and plastic wrap. He had packaged his contraband the night before and was in the bathroom hooping it up his anus. Once the check-out time came, a guard arrived to pick us up. We were separated and asked to leave the bags in the cabin.

Another prisoner had put out a *kite* (snitched) that Matt was going to be bringing drugs back into the prison. They held me in a room with Monika, and absolute terror surged through my body. *Oh, shit! We are busted.* They were in the cabin now searching my belongings; surely, they would find the hash bong, and I would be in trouble. I'm not sure if I've ever been that terrified in my life. My brother waited for me outside because he was my ride home. *What if I'm arrested? Will they let him take Monika? Oh god, what have I done?* The guards came back in, and I tried to remain calm; I couldn't believe my ears when they said I was free to go! My bags waited for me, along with my brother at the front desk. I could not wait to get out of there.

Matt didn't call me until the next day. He had been strip-searched and bent over for examination, but nothing was found. They kept him in a dry cell, hoping he would expel a package from his ass, but he held onto it until they finally let him go after twenty-four hours. The same guard protecting us must have been in the search party and taken care of the bags, letting me off the hook. He got his hash, steroids, and MDMA inside, and that was the last time I smuggled drugs into prison. Almost getting caught had scared me to the core. I realized I had put Monika at risk of losing her mother and would never take such a chance of jeopardizing my freedom again. It wasn't worth it. Funny how something can start out so simple and seem like it's not a big deal, then slowly start to snowball into something much larger and more dangerous.

I never imagined Matt's prison sentence would turn the both of us into criminals, and I never dreamed this Criminal University he attended was about to amp up its lessons. He had met some major players in there, and smuggling in all of the drugs was giving him the advantage of making good friends with criminals who admired his craftiness and ability to run drugs inside the prison.

One fellow in particular started grooming Matt for the cocaine trade. He wanted Matt to start moving large amounts of it for him once he was released from prison. Matt assured me this would be temporary, only to make some extra money to get us off to a good start. He told me it was a part-time thing and that he would still have a job. "Don't worry; I have it all figured out," he said. He often brushed my concerns aside; no one could tell him what he could or couldn't do. This could have been a great strength for him, but he always used it as a weakness.

He didn't tolerate anyone telling him anything, and it always landed him in trouble. I don't know why I stayed or why I went along with it all. My desire to have a family made me. He said all of the right things often enough to keep me tied to him, telling me he would take good care of us, that he loved us with everything that he had, and he was going to provide us with a great life. I wanted to believe him, so I did. I stayed and dreamed of better days.

9

Catch and Release

Just shy of two years after his sentencing, Matt was released on parole into a halfway house. Now, he could work during the day, visit us in the evening, and then return to the halfway house for the night. It was difficult having him leave every night, although the transition was probably best for both of us. It was hard adjusting to someone being in your space all of the time, no matter how loved they are.

Upon reflection, I'm so happy I had those first two years alone with Monika. It was a much more stable environment for her, and we had a beautiful bond. I nursed her until she was eight months old, and we went for walks with the dog twice every day, even in the dead of winter. Monika was absolutely adored, and I could give her my undivided attention. Right after she turned one, I started cleaning houses two days a week to earn some extra income. On the days that I cleaned, Monika stayed with Matt's aunt, who took excellent care of her. I socialized with a few friends during that time too. Jordy was in high school topping up her missing credits after years on the streets, and we stayed in touch. Kerry and I spent a lot of time together as she had started dating one of Matt's friends. Friffin and I were still friends; she had a baby the year before me and would often come over to spend the weekend. My life was very simple, other than my partner being locked away in prison.

After Matt moved home full time, we decided to rent a house in Markham, just northeast of Toronto. We rented the house together with my older brother; things had gone south between him and his fiancée, so he was selling his house and needed new living arrangements. He also had a business idea and knew Matt was the right person to help him get it off of the ground: growing marijuana. We found a bungalow and turned the bedroom in the basement apartment into the grow room, and my brother lived in the remainder of the apartment. Matt, Monika and I lived upstairs. My brother had the connections to get clones from a high-quality mother plant, and we bought all the equipment needed at a hydroponics store. We covered the bedroom from floor to ceiling with plastic to waterproof it. The windows were blacked out, and special growing lamps were fixed to the ceiling. We had around forty buckets all lined up with a watering system for easy feeding. Fans were placed around the room to create a natural breeze. It was exhilarating to get it going and watch the little clippings turn into full size, hearty plants. It was also very illegal.

Matt's parole officer came over to check out our new place, which was protocol, and I was terrified she was going to smell something or say she needed to inspect the entire house. I felt so much relief when she wrapped up the meeting after fifteen minutes of sitting in our living room and said that everything seemed great, and we could carry on!

Marijuana wasn't the only thing we were into. The only reason we could afford the increased rent on the house was because Matt had started selling cocaine. A relative took over the lease for our old apartment, and Matt paid the rent in exchange for using the place to stash the coke. He stored his product in the freezer and popped by when he needed to make deliveries. Matt also worked as a car parts delivery person in Markham; he needed to have a regular job to keep his parole officer happy. Eventually, his boss didn't need him anymore, but he asked to stay on and would work for free so he could maintain the front until parole was finished.

We started accumulating a lot of money, and we put a lot aside with plans to buy a house. I finally had my first car. We even bought into a tanning salon in Etobicoke with his buddy who got him into the larger-scale drug trade. I worked out with a personal trainer a few times per week and had gotten back into shape. Eventually, I wanted to start working again, so we put Monika in daycare when she was two, and I headed into the city to work at our tanning studio a few days per week. Even though we subsidized our life with drug money, we lived pretty normally with both of us working, going to the gym, and spending time with Monika.

I was devastated the first time I realized Matt was occasionally using cocaine. Since I had been sober for almost four years, I didn't want that back in my life. I thought he was crazy to take the chance of slipping back into a full-time addiction. Anytime I confronted him, he became furious and defensive. We had just gotten home from his buddy's wedding, and he went down to the laundry room, which was weird. I went down shortly after and found him cutting lines on our washing machine. Our new life wasn't so happily-ever-after.

Once the marijuana had matured, we clipped it, hung it to dry, and then bagged it. When it was time to sell it, my brother got greedy and tried to jack up the prices. Matt wanted to offload it all in a large quantity, which meant less money but also less work and money coming in fast. My brother had it in his head that he should be getting $15 per gram, which is ridiculous, and so they had a *huge* blowout. I didn't speak to my brother afterward for two years. He said Matt threatened to kill him; Matt said my brother was crazy and totally made that up. I wasn't there, and it didn't matter anyway: Matt was my partner, and if it meant losing a brother, then so be it.

Needless to say, my brother moved out, and we decided to purchase our first home. We had enough cash saved for a down payment, and one of Matt's friends was a crooked real estate agent who had connections to people who could make purchasing a house for two people with no real stability totally possible. They had fake documents made, and getting into our first home was as easy as stealing candy from a baby.

We found a great three-bedroom home in Maple, which was northwest of Toronto. I was twenty-two and Matt was twenty-four; Monika was three. I loved the house and the new neighbourhood. Shortly after moving, I quit working at the tanning salon. Money really rolled in from the cocaine business, anywhere from $20,000–$40,000 per month. Matt and I alternated driving vehicles depending on our moods; we had a Yukon Denali and a BMW M5 to choose from.

We had set a routine of heading to the gym separately but at the same time. Arriving there around 10 a.m., I put Monika into the daycare there for two hours, and we spent the morning working out together. Then he went to "work" for the afternoon doing his deliveries and was home by dinner. I always cooked, and he always made fun of me about what a terrible chef I was. It used to make me so angry and would often start fights since I believed I was a great cook, taking after my mother. I think he was so used to the traditional Polish meals his aunt made, so he'd scoff at my more Canadian-style meals: chilli, meatloaf, and pasta sauce with ground meat and veggies. Eventually, my skills developed further, and I'm currently working on a plant-based cookbook as I write this. To this day, I'm sensitive about my cooking being critiqued. I think I was traumatized by the mental abuse Matt would lay on me about my meals.

It wasn't only the meals: he was verbally abusive daily, often calling me bitch, slut, or worthless cunt. He was a monster. I believed he wasn't using; at least I tried to and turned a blind eye. Asking him constantly to quit selling drugs, I told him we had everything we needed now. "Let's quit while we are ahead."

But he kept telling me, "Not yet. Soon, I promise." Although I asked him to stop, a part of me didn't want him to. I loved having the endless amounts of cash to spend as I pleased. I went shopping and got my hair and nails done weekly, ate out, and got massages. We had a cleaning service at home and detailed our cars weekly. Money was never an issue. There was nothing I couldn't have, and I knew if he quit, that would all disappear. We lived life looking over our shoulders, always wondering if we were going to get busted. The friend we owned the tanning salon with, who was also a level up from Matt, had a thug come to his house and rob him at gunpoint. That scared me. No one knew where we lived, and we never had customers come to our house, but it was still a possibility, and it made me nervous.

We eventually had a run-in that shook us hard. Matt started to move kilos, a big step up from ounces and half-kilos. It meant more money, less work, and (we thought) less chance of getting caught as the number of people you're dealing with decreases. A friend of his from prison had a buddy who wanted to buy a kilo, and Matt had to deliver it to Montreal, Quebec. I had a really bad feeling about it and so did he. Money-hungry and eager to move up the ranks, he went anyway. One of his closest friends made the trip with him. They would spend the night and come back the following day.

I got a call from him later that evening, and he was shaken. He had been robbed at gunpoint: not only were the drugs stolen but so was our truck. The assholes took off in our SUV!

Matt and his friend took a long and expensive taxi ride home. It cost over $500. He was extremely upset, pissed off at himself for getting duped. I asked him if he had planned to retaliate. No, he wasn't; he said he was going to consider it paying his taxes and move on. It was a $30,000 mistake, a painful debt to repay. We still had to deal with the truck—where the fuck was it? Matt decided I needed to call the police and report the truck as stolen. *Say what? Hell no.* He really put me in some shitty situations occasionally.

"We don't have a choice. You're the least suspicious of the two of us—you have to call." So, I did. I called the police and told them I woke up in the morning, and my truck was missing. They came over and wrote up a report. I thought we were going to get busted for sure. Two days later, the police followed up and said our truck had been found, abandoned all the way in Montreal. They told me the window had been smashed in, and it was in line with a stolen vehicle. I couldn't believe it; at least those jerks had made it look like it was stolen. The cops told me it was being towed back, it would go straight into the shop, and insurance would cover everything from there.

Matt and I started partying again quite often on the weekends. I was only drinking and smoking pot, but eventually, we started using molly. We went out to clubs, boat cruises, or often to a friend's cottage. It wasn't long before one pill turned into twenty over a weekend. We got so fucked up that we were nearly paralyzed. Monika went to his mom's for the weekend who was so happy to have her, and we let loose. We started fighting a lot more, and it would often turn into all-out rage. He resorted to intimidating me, breaking things, and raging at me from the other side of a locked bathroom door. I would often take off to hide from him in there: his anger was terrifying. The fights were starting to happen all the time, and the drugs made it worse. We even worked out separately at the gym, though I still kept up with my healthy lifestyle during the week. I never missed workouts and adhered to a strict diet because my physical appearance was a high priority for me. I often hooked up with Jordy to work out. Eventually, I made a few new friends at the gym as well, one of whom would eventually become my best friend.

Eventually, Matt ended up back in jail. He failed a surprise urine test his parole officer asked for. He was locked up again for three months. The good thing was he went straight back into the minimum-security prison. I went up twice a week to visit him and ran the money for the cocaine business while he was away. He already had someone cutting and repressing the coke for him. They dealt it out to his customers, and I picked up the money. We had a money counter at home, and I had it counted and wrapped in $10,000 stacks with elastics. I drove out to Oakville to drop off the cash to his dealer, and everything ran without a hiccup while he was away.

When he got out, things went downhill really quickly. I knew we were in trouble when I picked him up from prison, and he had me drive straight to a pick-up spot to grab drugs. He was so good at brushing shit off. "Don't worry," he said, "I've just spent three months in prison. I want to have a little fun." I was pissed, but I knew there was no changing his mind, so I went with it.

A few weeks after he was back home, he proposed. We were in our master bathroom, and our soaker tub was full of warm bubbly water. I was already in the bath enjoying a glass of wine when he pulled out an engagement ring. There was no big surprise here: I had been pressing him to get married.

The ring was stunning: a solid two-carat diamond on white gold. I was delighted. After he slid it on my finger, he pulled out a little baggy of white powder. Cocaine. "No way! I'm not doing it. I can't go back to where I was. It's been so long; I've done so well. No," I said.

"C'mon, don't be such a party pooper. You're not going to have a problem. We are way past that. Just a little bit. Let's celebrate; we're engaged." I felt cornered, and I didn't want to ruin the moment by starting a fight. So, I thought, *Maybe he's right—I can handle it now. It's been such a long time; I can control it.*

He had already chopped lines on a magazine on the side of the tub. We each did a rail, and it was off to the races. I felt like a queen: my favourite high. So powerful.

We partied every weekend. Friday night, Saturday night, and even Sunday night. We were animals with it, and it never ran out because we had a never-ending supply. Matt and I started going to strip clubs and eventually got into ordering hookers. We dropped thousands of dollars every weekend on restaurants, bars, and women. Things were getting really out of control with our spending.

Our most outlandish purchase was a huge thirty-six-foot speed boat, and we rented a dock at a posh yacht club. We leased a third car: a Mercedes CL500 and even went on a few wild vacations. One, in particular, was to the Dominican Republic. Jordy came with us, and it was a shit show. We smuggled cocaine, crystal, and molly with us across the border. We wrapped it in plastic wrap, sealed it with a lighter, and Jordy and I hooped them in our vaginas. Scared shitless, we made it through airport security and had one wild week. After running out of cocaine, we managed to find someone there to buy from. They led us to a beach shack restaurant way off the beaten path; we were served up the biggest lobsters I've ever seen. Surrounded by palm trees and the ocean on a private beach, it felt like we were in heaven. Our last night, we stumbled along the beach to get back to the resort, and we bumped into a local who was lounging on one of the beach chairs. This was a giant man who had drunk himself into a stupor. He told us he was the night-time security for the resort and kept watch of the beach. Heavily under the influence ourselves, we got caught up in conversation with him until he stood up, and a gun fell out of his lap onto the sand. We wanted out of there! Scared shitless, we excused ourselves and took off as fast as we could. Jordy had been sober from cocaine for some time as well. That's why we brought the other drugs. Once she finished them, she got into the coke, too, breaking her sobriety from it. It was a major setback and disappointment for her.

Although things had started spiralling out of control, I was still planning a wedding. Getting back from the trip, I went into full planning mode. We were doing it very small, planning to have it in my mother's backyard. Jordy was going to be my maid of honour, and Monika would be the flower girl. Our guest list was only around thirty people. I sent invitations out six weeks before the September date.

Matt and I still struggled. The fighting was relentless, and the drugs and money were making us crazy. After one huge blowout, I'd had enough and said I was leaving. Taking off my ring and leaving it on the kitchen counter, I took Monika to my mom's for the weekend. I contemplated what to do. The thought of being alone scared me, and I also didn't want to lose the lifestyle. And though I had begun to really hate him, I didn't want anyone else to have him. I lost my vigour by the end of the weekend and went home to try to patch things up. He was very cold, and I could tell there had been a shift. I started to feel panicked. A few days later, he came home really late and went straight to the shower. I knew what that meant—that he'd had sex with another woman. Not because it had happened before but because I had heard that was something a man would do if he cheated. Matt never showered before bed. I felt everything unravelling, and I became desperate.

The next day, I went through his pockets, and I found tiny little clothespins, small enough to hang Barbie's clothes on. They had tiny pink bows on them. I could not figure out what they were for. I called Jordy, and she knew exactly where they were from. She had seen them at LaSenza, the lingerie store. *Fuck!* Losing my shit, I tore a strip off of him trying to get him to confess. He wouldn't budge and swore he met someone for business in the mall, and while waiting, he walked through that store and picked some up off of the counter and threw them in his pocket. *Liar. What a mess.* This was the end; we were going down in flames.

Desperately, I decided to try to reconnect one more time. Spending a day making a fancy meal of mussels and shrimp, I bought wine and a new piece of lingerie. I knew things were about to dissolve, and I didn't think I was ready to deal with it. That evening, I lit candles, got my sexy new outfit on, and waited for Matt to come home. I waited and waited and waited. He showed up around 11 p.m. and had zero interest in the food, wine, or me. I was crushed. He had always treated me like shit, called me names, and was physically abusive on multiple occasions, but he never rejected me the way he had done that night. My ego was crushed.

A few days later, he didn't come home. I called him, and he told me he was leaving for good. He asked me to pack his clothes and leave them at the front door, and he would be by the following day to pick them up. Shocked and devastated, I had to fall apart on the inside only. I didn't want Monika to realize something was wrong. She was a sweet little four-year-old who loved us both. While our lives had been wild, we had done a great job sheltering her from all of the craziness: we were both high-functioning addicts. Monika and I went to Canada's Wonderland that day. I needed her to be entertained and clueless as to how I felt. She had free rein to buy whatever she wanted: bracelets, paintings, pizza, and funnel cake. I couldn't believe my world was about to get turned upside down.

Matt and I spoke on the phone the following day after he picked up his stuff. He swore he hadn't met someone else; he had just had enough. I believed him because I needed to. The thought of being left for another woman was too devastating. After that call, he didn't take another call from me for over a month, and he didn't see Monika for four months. He even missed her first day of school.

Calling all of our friends to let them know the wedding had been called off was painful. I was humiliated. Later, I found out he had left me for a stripper who was ten years older than me and a single mom with her own child, one he would now be spending his days with instead of Monika. I hated her, and I hated him. It took a lot of years to let that shit go. Thinking back to how much I despised her and all the energy I wasted on hating her, I now thank her. I truly believe she was a guardian angel sent to save me from him and the toxic life we had lived. Today, I have so much gratitude toward this woman: she may have saved my life.

PART TWO

Shame

10

Fall from My Throne

Spending the first few months after Matt left waiting for him to come home was lonely. I was convinced he would miss me terribly, realize he couldn't live without me, and eventually come back. He never did. I spent my weekends drugged up on cocaine, out with friends, and avoiding my reality. My mind was full of fear, anger, and insecurity.

Monika started her first year of school, junior kindergarten, and when he didn't show up that day as he'd promised, I finally accepted it was over. I knew that if he couldn't show up for her, he was never going to show up for me. Now, I use this as an assessment of my relationships with friends and family. If people aren't capable of showing up for themselves, how are they possibly going to show up for anyone else? Taking expectations off of people saved me a lot of heartache. I expect to be treated respectfully and have good connections. Finally, I have come to understand that not everyone is capable of loving in the same capacity. Showing up in a relationship is the same. If someone has barriers to how much love they can let in or out, then their showing-up capabilities will appear in the same manner: a limited one.

Matt didn't show up. He failed and flopped miserably at co-parenting. I now understand his heart was closed, and he kept it that way as protection. He had been beaten down hard by life and chose to let it take him down. This was hard for a little girl to understand. My dear Monika, now twenty-one, understands his capabilities, though it will never erase the feelings of being a neglected child.

He married his new girlfriend within a year of being together and then did another stint in prison. At one time, he lived in Poland, evading the police. He eventually ruined that relationship as well, and it ended in divorce.

Once it was confirmed that Matt was really living with another woman, I put the house on the market. My home was beautifully kept, and it sold quickly. I purchased a condo in Richmond Hill, and moved in on Christmas Eve 2013. At twenty-three, I had no job or education; I was a single mom and addicted to drugs. Hanging on by a thread, I was unsure of where I would end up in life. Reinvesting the money I had was a smart move. Had it stayed in my bank account, it would have gone straight up my nose.

Money started getting tight. Matt gave me $1,500 a month the first few months after he left and kept up with all of the household expenses.

One day, my debit card was declined at the grocery store, and I knew then and there I was about to fall off my throne. There should have been $10,000 in our joint account; I usually was the only one using it. I trusted it was going to stay that way and hadn't changed it yet to a personal account. After calling him, he explained he was going to put the money back. He promised he was only borrowing it. More lies to pile on top of all the rest.

I spent a lot of time with friends and stayed on point with my fitness regime. Looking to start a career, I enrolled in hair school at Marvel in Toronto on Yonge Street. I also had a new boyfriend. We met at the gym; he was handsome, fit, and wanted to show me a good time. J and I dated for the few months leading up to my move into the condo, and he eventually moved in with us.

I dropped out of hair school within a few months as soon as we got to styling actual customers' hair upstairs at their salon. It felt so unnatural for me, and I knew I wouldn't survive in a hair salon. I immediately started working on becoming a certified personal trainer. Working out was a passion, I was fit, and I felt super confident in the gym. I quickly got a job at Extreme Fitness in Thornhill; it was only a ten-minute drive from my new place.

The child support from Matt dwindled to $750 as soon as I moved in with my boyfriend, and within a few months, it disappeared completely. I had a big mortgage, along with condo fees. The lease was done on my Yukon Denali, and it had to be returned to the dealership, leaving me without a vehicle. I hounded Matt after I had to return the truck, and he wasn't giving me any money. His response was to set me up with an old Honda Civic. He told me where it would be parked and said the keys were in it. I went to pick it up, and it was truly the oldest vehicle I'd ever been in, and I grew up in a family that only bought used cars. I started it up, got it going onto the main road, and it died! I left that heap of junk right there on the side of the road. My friend who had driven me down wasn't too far and came back to get me. I was livid and wanted Matt to suffer, just like I was. Now, I understand that he was suffering. No one just gets up and walks away from their family unless they are suffering.

A friend of mine was ready to buy a new car and sold me their old Camaro. I paid $1,500 for it and drove it for almost a year until I could finally afford to lease my own brand new Honda Civic. This happened after I left my job at the gym to work at a large corporation. I was in their data processing unit/mailing center. It was a whole new world for me, but I really liked it there. I made some new friends and really started to straighten out my life. Of course, I started a fitness program there and even led up to 200 employees through a stretch break two times per day, which I was acknowledged for with an award. I was starting to feel like a somebody.

I was finally clean from drugs. It happened when a friend of mine from the gym confronted me about my drug use. I was still partying all weekend long while Monika stayed at Matt's mom's. I told the friend it wasn't a big deal, trying to brush it off. They weren't having it and really pressed me. I was showing up wasted and late every Monday morning back while working at the gym, looking dead tired, run-down with sores under my nose from the cocaine drip. "It's like you have a cold every weekend and then get over it by Wednesday." It was quite evident for anyone who had an eye for it. I confided in the friend and said I was using cocaine all weekend long, staying up Friday and Saturday night.

I will never forget the words that came out of his mouth, "You should be ashamed of yourself. You're a mother. You are supposed to be setting an example for your daughter!" It was a huge slap in the face and one I needed. These words were a powerful message that made me take the next steps in getting myself clean once and for all. I had already been seeing a therapist because my life was such a mess. Feeling incredibly depressed and fearful, I called up all of my friends and told them I wasn't hanging out anymore. Jordy and I had already parted ways; she was off to law school and needed to be at a distance from the partying, especially the kind that we were capable of.

My therapist diagnosed me with bipolar disorder and put me on medication. After six weeks, my life started to change. I had gained at least twenty pounds due to some pretty severe binge eating and middle-of-the-night bowls of cereal and cookies after I quit the cocaine cold turkey. The medication helped me get better control over my eating habits, reduced my anxiety immensely, and helped boost my confidence, which is how I landed the new job. I was so thankful to have regular hours. The gym wasn't cutting it, and I had also been working as a hostess at a high-end restaurant on Friday and Saturday nights, and it still wasn't paying the bills. Eventually, I had to sell the condo, and I moved in with Matt's mom for a few months. His mom and aunt were always defending his terrible life choices, and the situation was becoming quite toxic, so I moved back home again. This time, I maintained my employment and spent evenings and weekends with Monika. I felt like things were really starting to work out.

I desperately wanted to meet someone. I loved having a relationship, and I went on a lot of dates, had casual hook-ups, and went through brief stints with actual boyfriends. Often, I would daydream of having a loving husband, more children, and a house with a white picket fence. I started to recognize there were a lot of real losers out there, and I was having trouble attracting the right mate. Finished with the games, I decided to take a break from men, sex, dating, all of it. It was time to focus on Monika and myself.

Monika and I spent a lot of time with my best friend at this point. We were friends while I was using, but she was married with three young girls, and our lifestyles didn't really match. She had no clue I was using; though, near the end, she had her suspicions. Once I got clean, we started spending a lot of time together. Monika and I often spent the entire weekend over there. Our girls became cousins to each other. I felt like this friend was the sister I never had. We watched movies, celebrated birthdays, hung out by her pool, and bonded like crazy. Our friendship blossomed quickly, and we went through some tough times and amazing ones too. It's incredible how the right people can come into your life at just the right time. I needed someone outside of my two families to help guide me and show me how beautiful life could be. This friend, Thyra, was that person. Going out to concerts and clubs together was so fun, and we were able to totally let loose. We also baked and took the kids cottaging and to the beach. It was the perfect balance of having an exciting life of my own and also having quality family time with Monika. The memories I created with Thyra and her girls over the next few years were some of my happiest moments. Life was really starting to turn around.

11

The Secret

After taking an entire year away from dating to improve my mental and physical health, I felt ready to start looking for love. Having heard about a book called *The Secret*, I was really intrigued and picked it up. I started reading it in the evenings after Monika was tucked in for the night. The words really resonated with me, and I found the chapters on finances and relationships very influential.

Manifesting was a brand-new term for me. I had never heard of this before. The power of positive thought had never come across my path. I was wholly engrossed in the possibilities this book laid before me.

I decided to put the advice on relationships into my daily routine. Telling people close to me I had a husband, I was married with children, had a beautiful home, and was very successful became routine. I told people that, yes, I was married; I just hadn't met my husband yet. He was out there, and he loved me very much; I knew it. I would get goosebumps when I spoke the words out loud, and I believed it so sincerely that I would get genuinely excited. Talking about *The Secret* with anyone who would listen filled me up, and I worked on manifesting my dream life constantly.

My mother had always been quite pessimistic, and she would often say something like "ok, sure you are." On one occasion, after a remark like this, I decided to challenge her. I told her I was going to teach her how to manifest. We sat down in the living room, and I asked her to think of something she really wanted and believed she could have. At this time, iPods had just come out, and that's what she chose. I asked her to close her eyes and envision herself holding an iPod, to feel it in her hands, and believe that it was hers. She went along with it and set the manifestation.

Later that day, Monika returned from her dad's mom, Maya and brought home with her a garbage bag full of clothes and items from one of Maya's wealthy clients. This was very common because her clients were always sending gently used, high-quality hand-me-downs for Monika. I opened the bag and sifted through, and guess what was inside? Not one but two iPods! Even I was shocked! I felt like the universe really had my back there, proving there was an abundance of wealth waiting to be attracted. My mother was impressed, but this didn't change her outlook on life.

I worked out regularly at the Good Life Fitness at Hillcrest Mall, which was near my house. It was the same mall where I had held down my first real job while pregnant with Monika seven years earlier. One day, I bumped into a gym friend I hadn't seen in a while. We were quite chatty over the summer, but then our workout schedules must have misaligned over the fall because I hadn't seen him in months. Over the next two weeks, we bumped into each other every time I was there, and he was really growing on me. I looked forward to seeing him each time I was headed to the gym. On one visit, he told me about his snowboarding adventures. My ears perked right up as I had grown up skiing and really wanted to try snowboarding. I told him we should go together sometime, and he responded with "yeah, for sure!"

Then, I asked, "How about this Friday?" I wasn't letting this opportunity slip away. He had me really excited to spend more time with him; Jon was really funny, entertaining, handsome, and fit. So, we set our date for that Friday. I told him I would leave my number at the front desk of the gym for him (this was before you carried a cell phone around everywhere). My heart and mind cheerily skipped home; I was so excited to have a date. It had been a year of celibacy, and I was ready to take the plunge with the right person. Could this possibly be the one?

I told my mom about Jon as soon as I got home: how we had been speaking for a few months and how something finally clicked. And now, we were going on this awesome and exciting date. Then, it hit me hard. I forgot to leave my number at the front desk!

The next day after work, I headed to the gym and prayed he would be there. I went to the elliptical machine to warm up as usual. After twenty minutes, I saw him walk through the door, and I immediately started flagging him down, like a crazy chick out of a movie. He never thought I was crazy, though. Jon had a great smile for me, and I explained I forgot to leave the number. He told me he was pretty embarrassed when he asked the receptionist for the number that Deirdre, the blonde girl, had left for him. She had looked at him with a face that said, *Yeah, sure she did, buddy!*

Jon picked me up at four o'clock on Friday afternoon. I was all ready with my Prada ski suit on I had bought a few years before when I was with Matt, who was an avid skier. Monika was as well—she had been on skis since she was two. I didn't have gloves or a hat, so I borrowed Monika's! The hat was knitted from navy blue yarn and had pink piping with a monkey face and ears. The mittens matched, and although it was juvenile, I wore them with confidence. Monika, Jon, and I look back on this now, and I could pee my pants with laughter at the thought. Turned out, my ski suit wasn't water-resistant, and neither were the mittens. It also turned out that I spent a lot of time falling when I learned how to snowboard, regardless of how much skiing I'd done. Jon was a real gentleman. He purchased a private one-hour lesson for me, and that really helped me get going. I was soaked by the end, but also had really taken to it and looked forward to the next time we would go.

On the way home, we stopped to eat at Kelsey's. We shared an appetizer, and each of us had a Sonoma salad—I loved those back in the day! The conversation flowed easily, and it felt so refreshing to finally hear someone speak from their heart. He was so honest about his goals in life and what he was looking for in a relationship. So many of our ideas aligned, like marriage, kids, and what we wanted in our lives.

I went home that night feeling on top of the world.

Our next date was a few nights later on December 21, 2007. We went down to Nathan Phillips Square in Toronto to go skating. The evening was perfect, the weather was mild, and the snow was gently falling down. It was truly picturesque. As I glided around in circles holding hands with Jon, I thought it felt just like the movies. I'm sure my smile went from ear to ear, and I will never forget the way I felt or how beautiful that evening was. It was only the second date, but I knew I was falling in love. We finished off the evening at a restaurant called Panorama that was on one of the top floors of a building with a beautiful view of Toronto. The night was magical; he had put real effort into our date, and it didn't go unnoticed.

Back then, I always celebrated Christmas Eve with Maya and her sister, who were still very involved in my life. Then, I celebrated Christmas Day with my family. It was important to me for Monika to have a relationship with her paternal side of the family, especially because they wanted a relationship with her. Holidays with them usually involved fighting, verbal assaults, and swearing. This Christmas promised to be no different, mainly because Matt had just been released from prison for the third time and was living with his mom. Monika hadn't seen him for almost a full year, so I agreed to pick him up from wherever he was to take him to Maya's. I was so far away from having any respect for him, but my guilt of knowing Monika wanted to know her father made me do it. Of course, his first request upon entering my car that night was to stop at the liquor store. I nodded to myself, confirming I knew what he was all about.

We made our way to his mother's in Richmond Hill, and upon arriving, his three aunts and an uncle by marriage were already waiting for us. The screaming and accusations began as soon as they saw he had booze. *This is going to be a fun night*, I thought. They fought off and on and moved in and out of speaking Polish and English. After ten years around them, I could usually understand enough of the Polish to understand what they had said. It used to really bother me, and I felt left out, but eventually, when I realized how much fighting they were doing, I didn't want in on the conversations anyway.

After dinner was over, I realized that Monika, who was eight at the time, and Matt weren't with everyone, so I went down to the basement to check on them, and I heard her saying, "Ok, no problem, Daddy."

I asked her, "No problem with what?"

She responded, "Daddy needs to borrow my Christmas money." *Say What? Hell no!* I could not believe this guy was trying to steal her Christmas money. Knowing he would never pay it back because he hadn't given her a dollar in years, I was furious. I told her absolutely not, and by this time, everyone had come downstairs to see what the commotion was.

Everyone got upset with him, and he lost it. He started yelling and swearing, telling us we were all fucked up. The uncle, who is half his size, tried to stand up to him, but Matt intimidated him quickly. I got Monika ready to go, and we hurried out of there. It never failed; he always ruined everything with his selfishness. I thought to myself for the hundredth time, *I can't wait until Monika is eighteen so I don't have to deal with him.* After getting Monika home and into bed, Jon dropped by on his way home from his family get-together. It was so nice to see him, and the disaster of my evening washed away while I cuddled in his arms.

Later that week, Jon surprised me with a snowboard and boots! I was floored with his generosity. We headed out snowboarding a few times over the following two weeks, and I progressed very quickly. Jon had a trip to Whistler planned in early January for a week of boarding, and he invited me to come along! Only three weeks after our first date, we went on one of the most romantic trips. The snow was falling nonstop, and every time we went downhill, it was on fresh snow. We had the most beautiful dinners out together in cozy, cabin-like restaurants. Anywhere we went there was a wood fire burning, enhancing the romance and mirroring back the fire blazing in our own hearts. One evening, driving back to our cottage, the snowflakes looked as big as my hand. It was absolutely magical. We came back from that trip deeply attached to each other.

Over the next few months, it was a dating whirlwind: restaurants, presents, and little weekend getaways. Jon swept me off my feet—with intention. He met Monika, and they got along really well. Jon was happy for us all to go out to the movies, shopping, or to indoor entertainment venues.

I finally got to see what a real, intimate relationship was like. Would I be able to keep my past in the past? What if he found out some of my deepest secrets? I vowed to bury them deep and leave them there. Some things were best kept hidden.

12

A New Life

My new life was well underway. Work was going really well, and I was happy there. I had started a lunchtime fitness program twice a week and led a ten-minute stretch break twice per day: once in the morning and once in the afternoon that up to 200 employees attended. Receiving an award for my role in creating a healthier work environment was very affirming; sick days and work-related injuries had gone down. They started calling me the fitness girl.

After work, I headed to the gym, usually meeting up with Jon for a workout, then home to meet Monika for dinner. Monika struggled a bit in school. Math was not her strong point, and we usually had homework to work on in the evenings. She was excelling at sports, drama, and English. A social butterfly, she was friends with everyone in her class. I felt like things were good. She seemed well adjusted, even though life had been rough for the first few years. Her father was barely in her life again, and I hoped the good example Jon was setting as a male role model would be her new example.

The truth always comes out, and this rung true for me the day Jon questioned me about my anxiety. He knew I was on medication and that I had been diagnosed as having mild bipolar disorder, most likely from the drugs or early sexual assaults. Jon felt there was more to it, however, and intuitively knew I was holding something back. He had already opened up about some of his own unsavoury behaviours; he was a recovered alcoholic and was six years sober after attending AA religiously. Jon had also gotten deep into cocaine use for a few years when things really spiralled out of control. I felt like I could trust him with everything, though I believe I would have held out without his push for me to tell him my story.

We had parked somewhere, hanging out and drinking coffee in the car, when I told him about my year as a prostitute. He didn't look disgusted or upset. Jon was genuinely curious as to what it had been like and was sensitive with his questions. I couldn't believe I had opened up about this; I thought this was a secret I would have to take to my grave. Had I really met someone who could accept all of me? The good, the bad, and the embarrassing?

He didn't flinch, and it did not affect our relationship in the least. I felt so loved and so safe for the first time in my life.

It wasn't long after that we started talking about moving in together. Jon still lived at home with his parents. He was running a small property management company from his bedroom there. Jon was responsible for around forty properties and also had his real estate license and was getting deep into the market. I wanted to move in with him, but I told him we had to wait until we were getting married. Monika had already been shuffled around too much, and I needed to be sure she was going into a stable environment. This sparked the idea of getting married and really starting our lives together.

A few months later, Jon had planned a surprise trip to New York City for us. I had never been, and I was really excited! It was July, and we had been dating for six months. I wondered if he might propose, but knowing how young our relationship was, I didn't get my hopes up too high.

We arrived at Trump Tower that overlooked Central Park, and I was very impressed. This was Jon's typical style: go big! He always went the extra mile when planning a date or a trip because he wanted everything to be perfect and memorable. Memorable, it was.

We arrived early, so we left our bags with the concierge and headed into Central Park. We walked to the lake, rented a rowboat, and rowed out to the middle of the lake. Looking around, I saw so many monuments I recognized from all of the romantic comedies I'd seen. Wow, I was totally lovestruck. Then, he got down on one knee in the rowboat and pulled out a tiny navy blue box. He popped it open and asked me to marry him!

I remember feeling a sense of panic thinking about how to respond. My answer was absolutely *yes!* The moment felt so perfect that it almost paralyzed me. I stood up, I raised my arms, and I said, "Yes, of course, I will marry you!" He looked a bit startled and asked me to sit down; that's when I remembered we were in a tipsy little boat, and I obliged quickly. I glanced around again to take in the view and marvelled at the romance of it all. Jon still looked unsure and asked if I liked the ring. *What's not to like?* It was a gorgeous two-carat single diamond sitting on a white gold band. I told him I loved it and that I loved him; I would have been happy with anything as long as we were together.

He smiled, and we kissed. Then, he started to row us back to shore, and I noticed the boat was not his cup of tea. Where we docked, there was a beautiful little restaurant overlooking the lake, and we stopped there to have lunch and celebrate. It was a full house, and they had to squeeze us in. We were so grateful and explained we had just gotten engaged and let

the host know how meaningful it was that they accommo-
dated us. Over lunch, the tears flowed. I thought of Monika
and how lucky she was to have this decent man in her life
as well. That's when he told me he had taken her to buy the
ring and that she knew he had brought me here to propose!
Could this get any better? I felt like Cinderella.

When we got home, we quickly started talking about
moving in together and decided to buy. I had money saved
from the sale of my condo the year prior, and Jon would
have made a good commission on purchasing our home to
add to the down payment. Both of our parents urged us to
be careful of the other, worried we were moving too quickly.
Nothing was going to stop us; we were full steam ahead in
planning our life together.

We found a three-bedroom townhouse in Richmond Hill,
and by September of 2008, we had moved in as a family. This
was Jon's first time living out on his own, and he felt the
pressure immediately. I made a modest income at my office
job and had some vicious beauty expenses. These included
a weekly blow-dry at the hair salon, weekly manicure, bi-
weekly pedicures, and a few hundred dollars per month on
skincare and make-up. It didn't take long before we started
fighting over money. We were both big spenders, him even
more so than myself. Custom suits and shirts tailored in
Yorkville, $1,000 dress shoes (he had up to twelve pairs),
and expensive trips. We easily dropped $15,000 on a week's
vacation. Jon and I both had a terrible case of "I deserve this.
Buy now—pay later."

Wedding plans started, and Jon and I paid for most of it
on our own. His parents were financially dependent on him,
which drove me nuts and was a huge trigger for full-blown
fights between us. The arguments got so nasty that the sub-
ject had to be put to bed. I realized he couldn't accept that
his parents were taking advantage of him at that time and

decided to bite my tongue. If he was happy with the way their relationship was, I would have to accept it. We had everything we needed, and if there was extra money he wanted them to have because he believed he owed it to them, then so be it.

I had been promoted to the legal department at head office, which added twenty minutes to my commute in both directions, turning it into an hour drive each way. It was a drastic change, and I didn't adjust well. I went from over two hundred employees surrounding me, continually interacting, to a department of ten people who hid in their cubicles all day. No more lunchtime fitness classes and no stretch breaks. I felt completely isolated. Feeling guilty for hating my job, as I knew it was an excellent opportunity to move up within the company, made it difficult to leave.

They had a great pension, full health and dental coverage, and good vacation pay. But all I could see was a trap. I felt like if I stayed, I was sentencing myself to prison. A permanent position was posted in my department, and everyone expected me to apply. There was another young lady I worked with who was a single mother and way more qualified than myself. Feelings of guilt arose knowing that if I applied, I would most likely get the position because I had connections higher up in the company. I knew she deserved it way more than I did and was much more qualified. Knowing this was not a long-term position for me, how could I take this away from her? I was tangled up inside, and I knew I needed to make a change. Sitting at my desk one day, I thought to myself that I wanted to smash my head right into my computer because I found the work so mind-numbing. Staying there wasn't an option. I went home to talk to Jon about quitting my job and getting back into personal training. He wasn't very supportive of the idea.

Jon didn't agree with it but told me to do what I felt I needed to do. I went to work the next day and gave my notice.

I was on top of the world, so excited to start up my PT business. Jon was visibly not happy with it, but I was determined to prove him wrong. I set up an in-home training business, where I brought equipment to my clients' homes for our sessions. Also adding in a few days working at the Extreme Fitness to top up my income. I was so happy to engage with people again. Still struggling with my finances, Jon blamed it on me quitting my job, though overall, I made a similar income. For me, the happiness was worth it. Meanwhile, our wedding plans were in full swing, and the tension with his parents was too.

His parents didn't want anything to do with our wedding. It was like pulling teeth to get them to participate in anything going on. I really felt like they didn't like me. Looking back now, I can see this was most likely because they knew they were going to be losing control of Jon, which eventually they did, though it took years.

His mom had a talk with me a week before the wedding to let me know she wasn't sure if she trusted me and wasn't sure if I was going to be good to her son. This was a few weeks after she told me I shouldn't trust him and should hide money away to look out for myself. I really tried to get into his mom's good graces. Inviting her to go get pedicures or dress shopping was always met with her scoffing at me, "Why would I buy a dress? I have perfectly good dresses at home." That wasn't the point; I wanted to spend time together. Continuing to envision us having a loving relationship I went to her belly dancing class to show her how interested I was in forming a bond. Pedicure together? No. Cake tasting? No. She didn't want anything to do with me.

Her sister came to visit to attend our wedding, and she asked me to host them all for dinner two nights before the wedding! I couldn't believe her nerve. She had never invited me to her house for dinner, yet had been to mine multiple times, and wanted me to entertain right before my wedding. I know she wanted to show off to her family how well Jon and I were doing, so I went with it. She asked me to do this entertaining right after she accused me of not being trusted as a wife, and I am now able to see the manipulation. My soon to be mother-in-law knew she would get her way if she made me feel insecure. I wanted her to like me so much and was deeply hurt they weren't accepting me into their family.

My wedding day still remains one of the happiest days of my life. I had the perfect wedding dress that fit me like a glove without alteration; it was also the first dress I tried on. My best friend was my maid of honour, and her daughters, along with Monika, were the bridesmaids. Jon's brother was his best man. I walked down the aisle with a huge smile on my face. In fact, I smiled all day and night, and my cheeks hurt by the time we got to dessert. We stayed in a fancy hotel in Toronto and had a couple's massage booked for the next morning. After going through our cards, I noticed his parents didn't give us a card and mentioned it to Jon, thinking they had possibly given it to him privately.

"No," he said, "they didn't give me anything."

I found this very strange. It came out later that his father told Jon's mother he had paid for our wedding! This was an outright lie; he hadn't given us a penny. He told his wife he had to sell their property in Newfoundland to pay for our wedding. The truth was that he sold the property to pay for his overdue income taxes. I was shocked at the level of manipulation they were capable of. This was only the beginning, though; I was about to uncover the high level of dysfunction in his family over the next few years.

The first year of our marriage was a blur. It started out with a fantastic honeymoon in Greece. We started out in Mikonos and finished in Santorini. It was pure magic, easily one of our favourite trips to date. Jon had been sober for many years by this time but decided to have only one drink on our holiday. I drank but always did when we were together, and he never minded or wanted to join me. We spoke about it, and I asked him to sleep on it. Wait one day, and if you still want to try it, then it's up to you. The next day came, and he still wanted to. And he did. We drank together for the remainder of the trip, and by the end, I saw the escalation develop quickly. In fact, on the last night, he didn't want to go to sleep at all, wanting instead to drink the night away.

We almost missed our flight early the next morning. On the flight home, he got extremely sick and swore he was never drinking again. He went straight back to AA the week we were home, and that lasted for a bit—until he decided he wanted to try it again. I was skeptical but didn't want to try to control him, so the drinking began again. It was weekends only at first. Over time, it spread from Thursday to Sunday night. He became moodier and was really nasty verbally at times. He never called me names but definitely gave off the vibe that he was more important than I was. Then, he would go the extreme opposite and spoil me with lavish gifts and write me love letters.

Over that first year, a lot of issues came up around his father, who had jumped into Jon's business as soon as it became profitable. He even started acting like he owned the company. Jon played along with it because he genuinely believed his father wanted to help him grow the business. I often pointed out inconsistencies with what his dad said compared to what he did (which was nothing), and this caused nasty fights between Jon and I. I was only looking out for my husband. Still, Jon wanted his father's adoration so desperately that he couldn't see past the manipulations. At this time, I remember thinking, *Holy shit, we are going to take care of his parents financially for the rest of their lives.* Looking back now, we can see that Jon started drinking to manage the stress because of his father. It was his way of coping.

I wanted to have kids right away so we could get that part of our lives going. By the end of our first year of marriage, I was pregnant. Jon wanted to wait, and this also caused a lot of tension between us. The pressure was high for him, and in some ways, this benefited us. Obviously, the stress was terrible for Jon, but it put our financial future into a great spot. Pressure of kids on the way, parents to provide for, and a wife and step-daughter to take care of had him working seventy hours each week. He was a machine; it's all he thought about, and I supported it 100%. There was never a time he was leaving the house at an odd hour that I wasn't waving him off with a smile. I had an expectation for how our life was going to be, and if it meant he worked like that, then so be it.

Charlize was born on June 10, 2011, and we had a home birth in a birthing tub. It was amazing; I was thrilled to be a new mom, and Jon absolutely adored her. However, he was emotionally unavailable due to the pressure at work, as well as being raised in an emotionally sterile environment, as I had. He didn't help me care for her at all, so we hired a part-time nanny so I could get a break a few times per week. Monika was twelve at this time, and she was a great helper. The two of us were still really close.

Jon's drinking had gotten out of hand, and he quit again when Charlize was a few months old. This was extremely hard on our marriage. A lot happened that year, and we had started couple's therapy to help us get through this tough time. Our three-bedroom house was beginning to feel small. We used one of the bedrooms as an office where my mother came in Monday–Friday, 9–5, to do secretarial work. And the company was ready to hire more staff. I had also gotten pregnant with our next baby; the two would only be thirteen months apart. We decided to buy a much bigger house and convert the basement into an office.

Jon and I found the perfect place. Even though it was outside of our budget, we decided to go for it. It was the best financial decision we made, as it would later lead us to early retirement. Our spending was still astronomical, and we had a few credit cards that we'd jacked up. The bank told us we needed to have them clear before closing, or we were going to have a problem. We hustled over the next four months to have everything completely paid down and succeeded with flying colours.

We were moving into my dream house: 4,500 square feet, five bedrooms, and fitted with only the best finishes. This move took us from Richmond Hill into Woodbridge; the two cities were around twenty-five minutes apart. It also meant Monika would be starting a new school for grade eight. We had no clue what kind of drama we were about to embark on, but shit was about to hit the fan.

13

The Struggle Is Real

The excitement built as we planned our move. With bridge financing in place, we owned both properties for a few days. We moved in right around Monika's thirteenth birthday and decided to let her have a big party in the basement of the empty house before moving in. Jon and I always tried to give Monika the world to make up for her biological father being absent from her life.

We had our good friend bring over sound and light equipment, bought decorations, and set up folding tables and chairs. We put way too much pizza and candy out. The night started out okay: the kids mingled, and some danced. I was eight months pregnant at this time, and Charlize was about to turn one.

Eventually, we had to shut the party down because a few of the boys got into a fistfight. As all the kids started to trickle out of our home, we realized this wasn't the most savoury group. It was the first little red flag that things may not be okay for our precious girl. I didn't want to see it or believe it, so I brushed it off as a one-time issue. Jon wasn't so convinced.

A few days later, we moved. The house had been freshly painted, new custom drapes had been installed, and we ordered a few new beautiful pieces of furniture from Restoration Hardware and Ethan Allen. The house came together quickly, and we organized it in no time. Two weeks later, I planned to host Charlize's first birthday party. The party was going to be on Sunday, so I spent Saturday morning shopping at Walmart for supplies, and then I stopped at Costco in the afternoon. I had so much on my mind that I put my cell phone down somewhere while at Walmart. It was a brand-new iPhone, only weeks old, and I couldn't remember where I'd left it. I only realized I had lost it when I stopped at home between the two stores. *Shitty.* I needed to keep moving, though, to get everything done. I went back to Walmart and re-stepped my way through with no luck, and customer service hadn't had anything turned in either. Totally irritated with myself, I headed to Costco. Because it was a Saturday, the place was packed. I had to park my car in the farthest spot away, which wasn't a problem until I left the store with my overflowing cart. I was two weeks away from my due date with baby number three, and pushing that cart across the lot is something I will never forget. I was exhausted when I got home, and after unloading the groceries, I told Monika I wasn't feeling great and needed to go lie down.

When I went up to rest, I couldn't get comfortable, always having the urge to sit up. Finally, after an hour of this, I started getting cramps. I was in full-blown labour. We had this baby at home as well, though I opted for a doggy-style position on the bed instead of the birthing tub this time around. Monika had called Jon and my best friend, who both got to me very quickly. The midwives came over, and in under six hours, baby Jonathan was born.

The only problem was that I had twenty guests coming over the next day for a party and no phone to cancel the plans! Luckily, I'd saved all of my contacts on our computer, and my best friend called everyone to let them know the party would be postponed by one week. The good part was that we had enough prepared food to get us through the week. My mother stayed with us that first week, which was really nice. She was retired by this point, and they had moved closer to Niagara Falls, which was about an hour and a half away. This period was probably the most love and affection I had felt from my mother; I'm happy we experienced it together. There is nothing like a newborn baby to bring a family together.

The following week, we hosted Charlize's birthday party. It was so lovely to have our friends and family over to celebrate her, as well as meet our newest addition to the family: baby Jonathan. It seemed the more stress I was under, the better I performed.

By this time, we had hired a full-time, live-in nanny. Jon still worked crazy hours and didn't have time to help much with the kids. Monika was now thirteen and wanted to be driven around everywhere: the movies, the mall, and to friends' houses. It felt endless, the shuffling between the teenage world and the baby world.

Jon still made a big effort with Monika as well. He feared she would feel left out with everyone else's attention on the two babies. Spending a lot of his free time with Monika was a top priority for him. It was vital to Jon that she didn't feel less than her siblings. We have generally been successful with this, except we were up against a strong opposing force as well.

Monika's other family. They were terrified she would choose Jon over her own father, or over them, and set out to ensure that never happened. They had two weapons: money and words.

Let's start with money. Monika was very spoiled by them, but at the time, I never saw this as a problem. I was pleased not to have to buy her everything all the time, so I was okay with it. She always had the newest iPhone, iPad, computer, shoes, and expensive coats. They paid for her nails or hair, an expense that escalated over the years. I believed this was their way of offering support since her father wasn't paying child support. Maya wanted to make sure the money was going directly to Monika and wanted her to know it. They often threatened to take gifts back or not buy her anything if she didn't do exactly what they wanted. It was clear manipulation, but they had been present her entire life, and making a big change would have been difficult and complicated: they wouldn't go away easily. We told her she didn't have to see them; it was her choice. But she liked the gifts, felt a connection to them, and put up with the toxic behaviour. Her relationship with them often had me in turmoil as I knew they were manipulative in a masterful way. I had once been their victim.

By this time, I was no longer in contact with them other than the occasional text. Their strong-handed parenting or life advice was of no interest to me any longer, and I kept them at a distance.

After they had called Monika and her friend prostitutes and stupid, we pressured her to cut them off entirely. Our family therapist had agreed as well. It was devastating to me to know they were so verbally abusive. Eventually, Monika called them to come to pick her up after we'd had a fight, and their relationship carried on.

Monika was very good at playing both sides against each other. Everyone had so much guilt over her father issues that she had us all wrapped around her finger. Their verbal abuse and manipulation came on strong. Often, they told her Jon and I didn't love her as much as our other children. They even told her we didn't love her at all. She still wanted to keep the relationship, though. It was infuriating that they would hurt her so deeply for their own benefit; it was unforgivable.

School started that September, and everything went well for the first few weeks. It was a big adjustment for Monika, who had only attended one school for the last seven years. Grade eight is tough anyway. With all of these kids turning into teenagers, hormones and egos ran high.

After those first few smooth weeks, some of the girls started picking on her. I think they were all picking on each other, really, but eventually, Monika couldn't take it. She started having severe anxiety about going to school. Monika came home at lunch and begged not to return. It was heart-wrenching for me. I so desperately wanted her to have a good experience and feel a sense of belonging, something I'd never had. We had multiple meetings with the principal and vice-principal, but nothing got better.

Eventually, Monika started to cut herself. I never knew a sorrow so deep. Having experienced so much pain as an adolescent myself, it still didn't compare to watching my own child suffer. When the cutting got worse, we took her to the hospital, and she was admitted to the youth psych ward for a few days. After an assessment, they determined she wasn't suicidal, and there was nothing they could do further to help her. The program was useless. I felt like they were looking to me for the answers, and they basically just wished us luck. This sent me spiralling down into my own emptiness, feeling desperate and alone. There seemed to be no one I could trust or depend on; I even questioned Jon, as he was her stepfather. Did he really have her best interests at heart?

Monika had also started smoking marijuana and drinking alcohol. I was rapidly falling apart. Depression came on strong, deep, and dark for me. I sobbed myself to sleep every night, thinking of how much internal pain she had. My other two children were only eighteen months and six months, so the stress at home was high. Jon and I were at the end of our rope, continually fighting over Monika. We both began withdrawing from each other. I was entirely consumed by her and couldn't function.

We decided to put her back into her old school. I drove an hour round trip twice a day to get her there. This helped for a while, but the red flags were still high.

I eventually found out her dad had been smoking weed with her at age thirteen and had given her other drugs as she got older as well. We called the police and Children's Aid to help us keep him away from her, but again, I was left disappointed. Nobody did anything to help us. We told her she couldn't see her dad anymore, and she went ballistic. She started screaming, crying, and breaking things. Eventually, she curled up into a ball on the floor in the corner of the kitchen and kept sobbing. "I want my daddy." It was hopeless. The one thing she wanted, she could never have. He wasn't capable of giving her love and adoration. It was something he had never received growing up and unfortunately wasn't able to learn as an adult. Again, at the end of our rope, we called the police. They assessed her and determined she should go to the hospital. She was incoherent and clearly in a great deal of stress.

After she was admitted, I sat with Jon in the waiting room while she was with the psychiatrist, and I got a text from her father. She had been messaging him earlier to let him know shit was hitting the fan.

Matt: What's happening with Monika? Where are you?
Me: We are at the hospital. She seems to be having a mental breakdown.
Matt: I'm coming right away.

128

Me: No, I think it's better you don't. It seems she's struggling because you have never been in her life.

Matt: Exactly, she needs me. I'm what she needs. I'm going to take care of her now. Everything is going to be fine.

Me: Don't come.

He didn't come, of course. Monika spent the night at the hospital and returned home to us again with good wishes. I was terrified she was going to really harm herself, even possibly kill herself. My world continued to revolve around her.

The following week, when I went to pick her up from school, she wasn't there. All the kids had gone, and I waited for fifteen more minutes, but she never came out. I walked into the office and asked for her. They called down to her teacher, who said she had been dismissed after school as usual. I walked back out to my car to find a voice message left on my phone from her father. "Monika is coming to live with me; it's for the best."

In the background, I heard her say, "Yeah, it's for the best, Mommy." My heart dropped into my stomach. I completely froze. It was one of my worst nightmares come true—that she would choose him over me. My heart was crushed. I'd given her all my love, a safe space to share her dark secrets without judgement, and all my free time. It wasn't enough—where had I gone wrong? I couldn't compete with the invisible cord that connected Monika to her father. She was desperate for his love and thought it was the answer to her internal yearning.

I walked back into the principal's office, who was a woman I had known for years, and explained the situation. The advice she offered was to let her go. She explained that if I tried to force her to come home, the battle would continue. "You offer her calm and support. Let her see what's it's like on the other side. Take a break."

Surrender? I thought. *To him?*

Heading home with a heavy heart, I prepared for a long discussion with Jon. He urged me to let her go live with her father. We had two small children and a marriage on the edge. *When do we get to take a break?* We couldn't compete: they would buy her anything and allow her to do anything. They'd convinced her to go live with them. I knew he was right. The manipulation and gaslighting on the other side was something I couldn't fight. Only time and Monika's intention could heal that wound. Monika needed to come to an age where she saw everything clearly. She needed to see how much I loved her, see the lies they told her about me weren't true. Eventually, she'd realize they were manipulating the situation to gain control over her.

I called them and asked to speak to Monika, who came on the phone. Feeling extremely vulnerable, I asked her if this is what she really wanted. Yes, she was going to live with her dad and his mom.

Her dad had just been released from prison—again. I could foresee how this was going to go wrong.

"Okay, I'll drop off your belongings. Know that I love you, and we are always here if you want to come home," I said.

The nanny and I packed up everything. I shuttled four garbage bags of clothing over to her grandma's. Now, I was angry. *You want to live with them? Have fun*, I thought as I piled everything on their front porch.

It took me a few days to fully accept the situation. Surprisingly, I slowly started to feel better. My stress was reduced, and I wasn't crying all the time. Jon and I started spending more time together and talking on a deeper level. It was like the eggshells had been swept off the floor. There was a tremendous amount of guilt, but I knew that as long as they were in her life, there was nothing I could do. The ship had sailed on gaining full custody, and I knew they would fight me to the death. I had never gone for full custody because her dad was never interested in her: I didn't need it ... or so I thought.

Jon and I had taken up running together to reconnect, help me get over my depression, and get back in shape after the back-to-back pregnancies.

We hired a coach and met with her weekly to run intervals on a track. She was a pro triathlete and introduced us to the world of triathlons, eventually convincing us to buy bikes and take up swimming. This coach was a major influence on our lives and the direction we were heading. I had no clue at the time how deep I was about to get involved in sport.

Jon and I had a great time training together. We started seeing a swimming coach and going to indoor cycling classes. Our fitness was increasing, and we were finally starting to feel happy again. I finished my first triathlon in the summer of 2013 and was hooked. We started to ramp up our training and even planned a training camp vacation for the winter.

Monika now lived with only her grandma. Her father hooked up with a new girlfriend and moved out weeks after Monika had moved in, abandoning her again. She seemed happy enough staying with her grandma, who was great at appeasing her. All of Monika's friends from school lived nearby, as they were living in Richmond Hill near the school and our old house. Even one of her best friends lived only a street over from her. My relationship with her was strained, but I refused to get drawn back into the dysfunction. I made it very clear that she was loved and welcome to come back home but that there were rules to be followed: she had no interest.

Her grandmother planned to move to a small town about an hour away. Monika would start high school in a town where she knew no one.

They made the move, and Monika hated it. She was still cutting herself at this time. Consistently calling me crying, she told me she hated it there. My answer was always "you hate it anywhere there are rules."

It wasn't long before she was hospitalized again. This time for swallowing a bottle of Tylenol. She had strained her liver severely. They kept her in the children's mental health unit for two weeks. Again, they released her, saying, "There's nothing more we can do—good luck!" No one knew what to do with these struggling teens. They were clueless back when I needed help, and they are still clueless today, nearly thirty-five years later. What a disappointment.

One of Monika's great aunts, her grandma's sister, owned a condo in Toronto but was very sick and had moved in with another of their sisters. Maya and Monika moved into the condo so Monika could go to school in Toronto, hoping this would help her. It most definitely did not help. She ran wild, skipping school, smoking joints every day, drinking on the weekends, and hanging out with friends as messed up as her. Her father was in and out and addicted to drugs.

Any time she wasn't happy with how they treated her, she ran to me and tried to get me against them. I was already against them, but I wasn't playing the game any longer. When Monika was fifteen, I finally told her I'd had enough of the bullshit. Either straighten up, or we can't talk for a bit. I told her I was here if she were in danger or was ready to change, but I couldn't be drawn into the drama. Of course, the other side took this as their opportunity to tell her, "See? We told you your mother doesn't care." It broke my heart, but she needed tough love, and I had to be extreme one way because they were extreme the other way with overindulgence and lack of boundaries.

The highs and lows over the next few years were crazy. I had become an elite age group athlete in triathlon, almost always taking first place in my category and top ten overall. The two younger kids grew up happy and content. Jon and

I were deeply connected. We decided we would homeschool the two younger ones, as our own experiences in school were not favourable, and our experience with Monika in public school was no different.

Monika was troubled right up into age seventeen. We eventually helped her get a small business going, and she was very responsible for once in her life. I had my hopes high that she would be okay. *Would I?*

14

Fall Apart

In 2016, my husband hit a wall. He had quietly suffered his whole life with low self-worth due to being raised by dysfunctional parents. He had become responsible for them as an adult, and they knew which buttons to push to make him fearful.

Jon had experienced health anxiety for years, but it was in full force over the winter of that year. In January, we vacationed in Tucson, Arizona. He made a trip to the hospital there because he was positive he was having a heart attack. They did the full battery of tests, and the results showed it was anxiety. His fears were so jacked up from his father's manipulation that it was manifesting as a tight chest, pain, and difficulty breathing. On another occasion, our family doctor ran a full set of tests, including wearing a heart monitor for a few days. They found nothing, and it was clear he needed to make some changes in his life. Jon still worked seventy hours a week. He was also training for competitive cycling; that was where he got his stress relief. It wasn't enough, though, and I discovered cycling wasn't the only way he was dealing with stress.

One night while lying in bed, he broke down in tears. It was the first time I had ever seen him cry after ten years together. This wasn't just a few tears; it was uncontrollable sobbing. He told me he had been taking oxycodone every day for the last few months.

My heart broke for him. He was so ashamed of what he'd been doing; he seemed like a man who was losing everything. I wrapped my arms around him and said everything would be okay, that I loved him and believed in him.

This news really triggered me, and I had to keep my insecurities at bay to fully dedicate myself to my husband's mental health. All the crap with Monika's dad came up; all the lies he told swam around in my head. I knew this was a different situation, but a traumatized mind loves patterns, and I had to take charge of those thoughts to avoid a downward spiral into depression. Matt had always made me feel second place to the drugs, and those thoughts were pouring in about Jon. I wondered how he could lie to me and if I could really trust him. We just couldn't seem to get out from under the dark cloud that I carried with me from childhood. I was determined to turn this around.

We saw a doctor who specialized in opioid addiction, and Jon got into the program. He also got into therapy and started working on the issues he had with his dad. Together, we took a look at our lifestyle and decided to make a considerable change. We had a big mortgage on a two-million-dollar house, and we decided cutting that cord was the first way to create low stress. We had enough money in the house to go mortgage-free if we moved one hour north of the city. Jon could cut back on his workload and focus on what he really wanted in life, instead of plowing through and trying to make as much money as possible for us to afford our lifestyle. We were terrified and excited. Jon and I knew that having no mortgage was a huge step in getting us to where we wanted to be in a few years. We always planned on retiring young, in our forties, and this step seemed to be the smart move in getting us there.

Jon tried to resolve his issues with his father. Unfortunately, as soon as Jon put boundaries in place, his dad turned his back on Jon. To this day, they are not in contact, and it's been life-changing for Jon. He was really able to step into his power and become the ultimate version of himself.

We felt so empowered; we had a list of our goals and knocked them off one-by-one over the next few months.

Jon and I bought a beautiful wooded 1.5-acre lot in Oro-Medonte, just north of Barrie. A bungalow, it was much smaller than the house we were leaving, but it seemed perfect. Setting up bridge financing again so we owned both homes for two months gave us lots of room for all of the renovations. The new house was outfitted with new hardwood floors throughout, a new ceiling in the kitchen, and a kitchen island. We renovated the basement to create our workout room, bike room, and a workshop for Jon. Customizing the house exactly as we wanted it, my dream had always been to have a pool, and we dropped one of those in as well. We also put in a separate hot tub, a place I've relaxed alone or with the kids on many evenings before bed. It was stressful organizing it all, but it was so worth it: the house was perfect for us. I thought this meant that my perfect life would begin. We were in a fantastic place financially, and we owned two other properties that we rented out. Jon and I were both still sorting through our childhood issues, and we were healthy with beautiful children. Time to relax. For some reason, I couldn't relax; there was this constant knowledge that I was not okay. Emotionally and mentally, I was not okay.

In December of 2017, I was working out in the basement. I was doing an hour and a half workout of plyometric jumps, something I did weekly as a part of my cycling training. My cycling strength had really fallen back; I was tired all of the time, and I was really concerned about what my 2018 season was going to look like. This was going to be the second year of running my own women's team, HighGate Racing, of which Jon and I were the founders, and our property management company was the title sponsor. Of course, I put pressure on myself to be really strong and fit; I wanted to see how far I could push myself.

As I got halfway through that workout, I caught an angle of myself in the mirror that made me focus on my stomach. It looked so bloated. Stopping, I did a full-body scan in the mirror. I noticed that my arms and legs were looking lean but that my stomach seemed quite pudgy. *Well, you're almost forty. You've had three kids. Maybe this is when it starts to go. Maybe a flat tummy can't be maintained after a certain age,* I thought.

Continuing with my workout until I caught another glance of my stomach, I thought, *That looks like a potbelly. Potbelly? Pregnant belly? No. I can't be. It's impossible; I have an IUD. When was my last period?* I couldn't remember. I'd been so stressed with the move and renovations that I blamed everything on stress.

After I finished my workout, I quickly went upstairs. Jon and the kids were lounging in the living room, and I told him I was going to Shopper's Drug Mart to pick something up.

As soon as I came home, I went straight to the bathroom. The moment the pee hit the stick, I saw a + sign; no need to wait. I was very pregnant. Putting my head in my hands, I began to cry. This wasn't in the plan. We were getting close to our retirement. My kids were all out of the difficult toddler stage. My cycling would have to be put on hold. My body won't be mine for the duration of pregnancy and breastfeeding. This isn't a part of the plan.

I headed out to the living room, and Jon looked up. After telling him the news, we stared at each other in disbelief. We were both shocked: this wasn't part of the plan.

When I went to the doctor, he was very concerned about the IUD and strongly advised us to remove the IUD, which had a 40-50 % chance of ending the pregnancy. There were a lot of complications that could arise to endanger me. He sent us for an ultrasound: the baby was there, and so was the IUD. It had moved further into my uterus. The doctors weren't sure if the pregnancy moved it or if it had previously moved, and that was how I got pregnant. Regardless, even with it in a different position, I shouldn't have been able to get pregnant. The IUD was made of copper, which is toxic to sperm. The chances of pregnancy were less than 1%.

I was already twelve weeks pregnant and about to start my second trimester. Everything was so clear now: why my cycling was going downhill, all of the naps I was taking, the weight gain, tender breasts, no period. How could I have not known? It's really amazing how powerful our minds are. I was so convinced I couldn't get pregnant with an IUD. After using IUDs without issue for seventeen years combined, getting pregnant with one was just not on my radar, and I found other things on which to blame those symptoms.

My family doctor referred me to an OB-GYN for further consult. We went to the hospital, and she advised us to remove the IUD as well. I told her there was no way I was going to intentionally put my baby at risk of a miscarriage. She told me about all of the risks if I didn't remove it. The biggest concern was that an infection could start from the IUD piercing something, leading to a premature birth and high risk to myself with the infection. I didn't bat an eye and refused to do anything to jeopardize the baby. The baby

I'd never wanted was now irreplaceable to me. I would do anything to keep this pregnancy. The following few weeks carried a lot of tears. I was a wreck because I constantly worried he might not survive; the miscarriage rate was 40–50 %. It didn't seem like the chances were good either way. I waited, and I listened to my intuition. Something inside was letting me know everything would be okay.

I had to go for ultrasounds with a specialist every three weeks to make sure things still looked good. I convinced the midwives in my area to take me on as a client even though I was considered high risk. They made me agree to give birth in the hospital and that I would continue to see the specialist.

Along with this pregnancy came a deep depression. Jon and I had talked about having another baby, but because my postpartum depression was so bad after the last two, we didn't dare take a chance. I was expecting the postpartum depression to come with this one, but the prenatal depression was new to me. Giving up my cycling was extremely hard, and even though my fitness suffered due to the unknown pregnancy, I was still in great shape. Our lives revolved around it. We had to cancel three vacations we had planned for that winter. Because of the high risk of preterm labour, we couldn't take a chance, and we couldn't buy medical insurance for an unborn baby. I was crushed. We were used to spending four to eight weeks away over the winter, and now I was stuck.

I stopped going out and didn't see friends often. Canceling plans became normal, and I only left the house when I absolutely needed to. I was very good at putting on a mask around the kids, never letting my depression show around them. I hid my tears well, and because it was winter, it seemed totally normal to be holed up in the house.

One afternoon, I sat on the stairs leading down to the basement and suddenly felt so much panic. Completely caught in fear that I was never going to be good enough, that I was going to be trapped in this state of emotional chaos forever. I thought about suicide that day. Never intending it for myself, but I understood how someone could take their own life. When the voices in my head got too loud and too out of control, it tormented me. It felt like torture, and I knew I couldn't live with it forever.

The next day, Jon found me sobbing in our master bathroom. I told him I thought he and the kids would be better off without me. Feelings that I was a drain on the family were coming on strong. A burden. He couldn't believe what I was saying and with how much conviction I was saying it. I was our children's entire world. Since I homeschooled them, we were always together. They truly adored me, and I dedicated myself to them 100%. Depression distorted my perceptions, and I couldn't see reality. Jon had finally had enough of my darkness and urged me to get help. I said no; I told him I had received endless hours of therapy since I was eleven, and if I wasn't fixed by now, I was not fixable. He said, "Please, just try one more time?" Jon advised me to take my mental health on as my most important project and encouraged me to do one thing every day that was a step in the right direction. Baby steps would turn into miles over time.

The following day, I researched therapists in the area and booked an appointment to see someone. Feelings of hope and curiosity as to how the first session would go immerged. I sat tight for two weeks to get to that initial session. Upon meeting her, I was engulfed in a friendly and warm environment. I told her most of my story, and she was so warm and understanding. She made me believe I could move forward. I saw a massive amount of work and pain in front of me, but for the first time in a long time, I was motivated to do something about it.

In her waiting room, I saw a flyer for a women's support group led by my new therapist along with another therapist and asked what it was all about. She told me it was a group of ten women who didn't know each other, and they met once per week for a group therapy session. "Its amazing," she said, "you should try it." At that point, I was up for trying anything to get better. My baby was due in four months, and I needed to be in good mental health for his arrival and be prepared for the possible onset of PPD.

I was really nervous about being in a group. *What would it be like? What if the women judged me poorly?* With grace, I pushed my worries aside and showed up anyway. I'd been in worse situations. If I didn't like it, I wouldn't go back.

The following week, I followed through with the commitment and drove over to the location, the other therapist's home. As I walked up to the front door, I thought, *Holy fuck* as I entered, unsure of what would unfold ahead of me.

PART THREE

Wholehearted

15

Collective Healing

I entered the living room in the back of the house; they had arranged it to seat ten women comfortably on couches and chairs in a square. The room was brightly lit through multiple windows, and there was a very calming décor. It had a breezy oceanside feeling.

Late and already feeling uncomfortable about that, I sat down quickly in the last seat left. I was already worried they were judging me for being late, thinking, *I must look like I don't care about my mental health if I can't show up on time.* Thoughts like that always flew though my head: never measuring up, never enough. They went around the group, and everyone checked in and told a bit about whatever issues had arisen that week.

Then, they got to me. The therapist let me know I could pass, or I could share a bit about myself and why I was there. Always able to see opportunity, I knew this was a chance to get some emotional pain out of my body. I would most definitely not pass.

"Hello, my name is Deirdre. I'm 4.5 months pregnant with my fourth baby, and I'm depressed. I've suffered from post-partum depression with my other pregnancies. I've experienced a lot of trauma in my life. I feel like if anyone knew about my past, then they wouldn't like me or want to be my friend." I started by going through the major traumas of molestation, rape, prostitution, and drug addiction. Everything poured out of me in one big swoop. Now, after attending many different groups since, I saw that this was not the norm. Most people took months or even years to divulge that much intimate information. Time was not something I felt I had any longer. I needed to be well … now. My mental health had affected me my entire life. Sadness, loneliness, and depression had engulfed me since childhood. I could not bear the weight of it any longer; I could not raise my children to my optimum capability if I didn't get better.

Going back every week, I continued to divulge more and more. I shed so many tears, and I felt all of the feels. Some days were easy, and I could see the light. Other days were hard, and I felt vulnerable and broken. The most important thing I learned was acceptance. These women accepted my good days and my bad. They supported me through my ah-ha moments when everything came together and also on the days when I was scared, confused, and feeling like a failure. I never seemed to change in their eyes. They always thought I was special. These women taught me that I could view myself through the same lens.

Women empowering women was a new lesson for me. I never knew this existed. There had always been some type of competition between women in my experience. With these ladies, it was different. We were all willing to go to our own depths of vulnerability in front of each other, and this gave us our bond. Everyone cried tears of shame, sorrow, fear, and guilt. Recognizing our own pain in each other was truly remarkable for recovery. Seeing each other for exactly who we were—no masks, no pretending, just raw truth—was exactly the recipe for my healing.

During this time, my oldest daughter, Monika, had fallen off track. She was in an abusive relationship and making very poor decisions. I had helped her start up a small business and was expecting some of the money I had put forth to come back to me. Making her stand on her own feet and understand that handouts would not help her in the long run was a lesson she needed. Monika always felt entitled to my money for multiple reasons. The biggest problem was her dad's side of the family. His side always used money to show they loved her, and now this was what she expected from everyone. They also told her I didn't love her because I would make her pay me back money I had lent her. In a way, she had been brainwashed by these people to her own dismay.

Monika had broken up with this boyfriend, and I was so happy, thinking she was ready to start on a path of self-care. I was very disappointed when she told me she would be flying to Mexico to visit him. He was in Mexico because he had been deported from Canada.

I was furious, and I told her she better plan on paying me back my money before taking a vacation in Mexico. She went to Mexico, and I put boundaries in place that her and I would not speak unless she was in serious trouble with the law, in the hospital, or ready to make big changes in her life.

Standing up to Monika in this way was extremely difficult for me. The struggle between being too hard or too soft was real. I never knew if I was doing it right.

My group supported me through this decision. One lady in group was often quite quiet. She came up to me at the end of group the day I told them I was cutting Monika off and said, "Thank you for sharing your experiences with your daughter. I have a daughter that takes advantage of me and is using drugs. She's causing a lot of turmoil in the home, and hearing you gives me strength that I can stand up to my daughter too." I was so grateful for this exchange. Someone believed in what I was doing when I wasn't sure I believed in myself. This type of understanding is profound. That is the magic of a support group that is well run and well organized. You never know how surviving your own struggle is empowering another to overcome their own. You realize we are all struggling to get it right. Most of us cover it up well with our smiles and nods that reassure us that, yes, everything is okay.

Everything is not okay. We are all hurting. No matter how perfect of a place you get your life to, some shit is going to go down. Even now as I write this book, my life is set up exactly as I want it to be. We are on a five-month vacation between California and Arizona, we have financial freedom, and everyone is healthy, but I still have my oldest daughter walking the wrong path, and it breaks my heart. That's the shit. There is always going to be something right around the corner, ready to rain on your parade. What's new about how I handle it now is that I know I have a choice. I have a choice in how I'm going to react. Either I can decide to let it take me down that nasty hole of guilt and shame, or I can acknowledge it and say it's not my problem to carry anymore. I have the option to free myself.

Some days, I attended group, and I wouldn't have anything going on that week, so I would pass on my turn. Surprisingly, these days often come with great life lessons as well. Someone may bring something up that is going on in their own life that may stir something inside, and you realize you still have work to do.

As things wound down from attending that original group, I had a lot of healing done. I was in a great place to give birth to baby number four. My depression had let up, and I felt like my healthy self again.

The pregnancy had progressed without any difficulty. We kept knocking off the weeks, celebrating another week closer to a safe delivery date in case of premature labour. Well, he was going to make me wait all the way up to a day after the due date. On May 30, I went into labour at 12:30 in the afternoon. The weeks leading up to the delivery, I started having anxiety about delivering in the hospital. I felt safe at home; I know home birthing. The issue was that the midwives only worked with me because I had agreed to give birth in the hospital, which at the time, I meant. Now, I was having major second thoughts. My intuition screamed at me to have this baby at home. I brought it up a few weeks before delivery with my midwife, and she said they would not plan a homebirth, but they couldn't deny me care if I was in labour at home and refused to come into the hospital. I thought, *Perfect, then I'm having this baby at home.*

After my water broke, I called the midwife who said I should meet her at the hospital. I said, "No, I'm staying home." She was clearly distressed over it, but I wasn't backing down. I told her to come to my house, or I would be having the baby on my own with the help of my doula and husband. Three hours of labour later, Kayden was born, perfectly healthy at eight pounds three ounces. The IUD was delivered alongside my placenta, and all was well as I knew it would be.

We packed the placenta and had already pre arranged to have another doula pick it up to dehydrate it and have it put into pill form. I had heard from multiple sources that this was a great way to prevent post-partum depression, and I was willing to try anything. Guess what? I had no post-partum depression. Now I'm not sure if it was all of the work I had done on my mental health, the support system I had set up, or if it was the placenta pills. Maybe it was a combination of everything. I do know that it was amazing to spend the next year feeling good about myself and not struggling with my dark, inner demons.

In the fall, I joined the next group being put together by the same therapists. Two of the ladies were the same as the previous years, and everyone else was new. My experience was the same. I felt loved, supported, valued, and seen by these women. Some of us really bonded well, and when the sessions were done, instead of rejoining, we started our own group. A few of the ladies invited someone they new who needed support and would be a good fit. In the end, there were ten of us in total. We set a day and time that we would meet every week and committed to it. It's been one of the greatest blessings in my life. It is a true sisterhood. I have found the courage to write this book because of these new friends.

I also reunited with Jordy after almost fifteen years of separation. My oldest daughter asked me about her because she knew her through Matt. Jordy had worked as his lawyer a few times. We had spoken through email a few years back when I was trying to get Monika's passport updated, and her father was in prison. I had to take the forms into prison to have him sign them there. It was absolutely dreadful and definitely pulled me into my past. They are no longer in touch, and this made me feel safe reconnecting with her. She was in the process of writing out her life story as well, and we saw a lot of synchronicities in our lives. It took quite some time for the two of us to get caught up on fifteen years of history, and now it's as though we never had the break. We are now completely committed to supporting each other through the next phase of our lives. It's very crazy how that relationship came full circle. She definitely was an inspiration to my writing as well.

16

Courage

I now had a great support system in place. It was like nothing I had ever known in my life. My husband is my greatest supporter, but he's only one person, and he has a lot of his own big goals he wants to achieve and couldn't be expected to be my full-time cheerleader. With my new crew full of people old and new, I was really inspired to keep moving forward toward a calling. I had visions of sharing my story publicly through speech and writing. I wanted to get my healing journey out there to help others who were stuck or felt alone as I once did.

I believed in my healing through group therapy so much that I got connected to a local charity in my area so we could start more of these groups. Wanting more women to have this experience is a big goal for me. Getting it off of the ground is still a work in progress, but hopefully by the time this book is published, it's running full swing.

When I'm very direct with what I want in my life, things start falling into my lap. This happened to me during the summer of 2019. I had joined a plant-based dragon boat team that trained and raced in Barrie, Ontario, very close to my house. A friend of mine organized it, and I was committed to trying new things and getting back in shape after having Kayden. Plus, it was a great cause; fundraising went to help animal sanctuaries.

One evening after practice, our coach told us about a local event he was hosting. It was in a restaurant, and he had four speakers coming to tell a personal story. My ears perked up instantly. He told us he hosts it once per month and was always looking for speakers. I immediately stepped forward as everyone else stepped back. Raising my hand, I said, "I'll do it!"

He looked a bit surprised and said, "Okay, normally, I don't get people volunteering; I usually have to do a little convincing." I knew this was the universe opening a door for me, and I wasn't going to shy away. He put me in for the following month.

I hadn't done any type of public speaking since grade eight, and I was terrified at how I was going to memorize my speech. Speaking to my husband later that night, he remembered hearing about a program called Toastmasters. A quick Google search found three groups in my area. *Excellent*, I thought. I reached out and connected with the one that met on a day that worked best for me. In one week, I was going to start my public speaking classes!

This is what I love about universal energy. If you put your true desires out there and set intention, things will start to gravitate towards you. Often times when we start to get what we want, it can be terrifying!

Speaking and writing has completely terrified me. Having these new dreams and goals for myself has made me feel like an imposter. I often had thoughts like *who do you think you are?* Or *no one wants to read anything you write; you're a grade eight graduate.* I would never say something like this to a friend, yet I had no issue talking to myself this way. Viewing myself as my past self was still something I needed a lot of work on and quite possibly always will. I often remind myself I have experienced a lot of trauma in my lifetime. Of course I'm going to have these issues to work through. Anyone would, and it's totally okay. Learning to love and accept myself even though I'm not perfect has made me feel whole.

In fact, sharing my story bit by bit has really helped me sort out some of those issues. Connecting with others because of different stories I've shared when it resonates with them really broadened my perspective on how we all struggle. Young women thank me for being honest about disordered eating, and they let me know they don't feel so alone knowing I've struggled too. Men have shared their stories of sexual assault with me, and I can see how they struggle with it and often don't feel they have a safe space to talk about it. Women have opened up about their own experiences with sexual abuse and/ or rape, even when they've never told another person. I feel so blessed and honoured to hold space for these people, and they have no idea how much they help me. When they share with me, not only are they being courageous, but they are also increasing my courage for the next step on this journey.

I have carried so much shame, fear, and guilt. Honestly, I still do. The bright side is that it is drastically reduced, and I am now also able to switch that negative thinking; I talk myself out of those draining conversations with myself that I used to let control my mind. This is my dream for human-ity—that we all learn how to shift this shame and step into our true power. Vulnerability is key to harnessing this power. I don't think everyone needs to get up on a stage and spill all of their trauma; there are so many other ways to share. Support groups, therapists and trusted friends. After I went through all of those resources myself, I still felt like I needed more sharing, more Collective Healing.

I had my chance at the MoMonday's event my dragon boat coach hosted and had me all signed up for. After a few weeks of my Toastmasters classes, I started working on my speech for that evening, and the speech was called "Collective Healing." I practiced my speech in my Toastmaster's class, which really helped me combat my nerves.

The night of my speech at MoMondays, I was terrified. I couldn't believe I was going to get up in a room full of people and tell them I used to be a prostitute and drug addict. What was I thinking? Why did I have this obsessive need to get it out there? I always went back to think of who I might be helping. I told myself, *There is someone out there who needs to hear your story to help them recover. If everyone hates you after but one person says you've changed their life, then it was all worth it.*

I sweated profusely, even though I wore a tank top. Heading to the bathroom to run the dryer on my shirt every fifteen minutes added to the anxiety, and I'm not usually a sweaty person. I had just read Gabby Bernstien's book, *Super Attractor*, and she had great tips in there about how she managed her stress before a speaking event.

Finding a quiet space as she suggested, I spoke to the universe to ask for guidance and courage. I asked to be guided to help the community heal.

"Next up is Deirdre Maloney." I was called from the stage and off I went. My husband and his brother were there; most of the women in my support group were able to attend as well. A few members of Toastmasters and a few friends from cycling and dragon boat racing had come out to support me too. It was very humbling to have these amazing people there that night. I shared my story flawlessly and felt on top of the world when it was over. My friends and family oozed with pride, and I knew I had made the right choice in sharing my story publicly.

At the end of the night, the loveliest girl with one of the most beautiful smiles I've ever seen approached me and said, "Thank you so much for sharing your story. I have a similar one, and I needed to hear that. You were amazing, and I feel like I need to connect with you." I was blown-away. She was my person. If everyone in the room thought I was a horrible person, as I had feared, she was the one that made that ok. We exchanged information, and now she is one of my sisters. I am now so deeply connected to her, and I know the universe aligned us to give me that sign; *Yes, I am on the right path.* My brother-in-law left shortly after the speech; my husband walked him out to his car. When he came back in, he carried a beautiful arrangement of flowers his brother had brought for me. The most beautiful thing about the arrangement is that it had lilies in it. I had just finished the chapter in Gabby's book on spirituality. She spoke of lilies and said that if you are looking for a sign that you are on the right path and you come across lilies, then that is your sign. I was so grateful for this sign. It was the perfect ending to the evening.

Later that night, I was high from the major adrenaline rush doing something that scares the shit out of you gives you. My friend texted to check in and make sure I was okay after divulging all of my deepest, darkest secrets. *Oh yes,* I replied. *I'm fantastic—no problem here!*

The next day, I woke up in a complete panic and messaged my friend right away.

Me: OMG, what did I do? I told everyone I was a prostitute. Drug addict. Grade eight graduate! What is wrong with me? What was I thinking?
Friend: Sounds like you have a vulnerability hangover.
Me: OMG, it's really a thing!
Friend: Yes, your adrenaline shot up really high last night, and now you're crashing. Totally normal! Yes, it's a thing.

This friend and I are both really into Brene Brown and absolutely love her teachings. My friend spoke to me for over an hour on the phone, calming me down and going over all of the positivity from the previous, now dreaded, night. After that long conversation, I curled up on the couch and watched Brene's Netflix special, *Call to Courage*, for the third time.

I knew I had to sit in those uncomfortable emotions, and they would soon pass.

That afternoon, another friend helping me with the editing of this book messaged to see if she could drop by to work on the book proposal. I felt shitty, but I really wanted to get started on it, so I said yes. It forced me to get up and get dressed, clean the kitchen, and make tea. Once we started working on the book, I had a new spark of energy. I started feeling really excited about the idea of publishing a book, and all of my worries of not being enough finally dissolved, for that day anyway. Looking back, I now know the universe aligned this visit from my friend to give me yet another sign to keep moving forward.

I was ready to take the next step on this journey that I had such a clear vision for and hoped deeply it would come to fruition.

17

A Wholehearted Life

It's been a long road to arrive at this wholehearted life I'm living—a roller coaster of a ride with so many highs and lows. How did I ever stay afloat? Upon reflection, I can see the process of arriving to this place of peace has been a drawn out one. There is not one particular moment that was life changing. Instead, it was a multitude of small moments, baby steps that accumulated over time.

The most obvious change was getting sober from drugs fifteen years ago. That confrontation from someone I respected smacked me in the face with his brutal honesty and brought me into myself. Getting sober is not easy; it's mentally painful. You feel as though you are giving up your entire life, and in a way, you are. Dropping all of my friends and starting a new life was scary. Mental illness kicking in full throttle and not being able to self medicate sucked. I gave up one life, and in exchange, I started a new one. At the time, it didn't seem like a good trade. The drugs are such an intimate part of your life, and they seem irreplaceable. Intimacy is false; the drugs are taking away your capability to have true intimacy with yourself or anyone else. This is a struggle you need to wade through, and it's not easy. It is worthwhile, as I can now look back on all that I missed. The drugs covered me up; they helped me hide the pieces of myself I was terrified to uncover.

Getting sober for me included therapy. I've been to many therapists and group sessions and some have been much better than others. If it doesn't seem like a good fit, find another. We all click and find comfort in different ways. Don't expect your first therapist to be the end all. Going on medication for me was a huge turning point as well. This really levelled me out and helped me stay sober. Looking back, I can also see it stifled my creative side. I would highly recommend medication to anyone struggling; it could be the little push that you need to get to the next stage in your life. I am happy to say that after fourteen years on medication that worked well for me, I have now been off meds for one year and am thriving. Do not come off of medication without supervision. I am only writing my personal experience; this may not be the right path for you.

I also started using alternative medication. CBD and THC oil helped me manage my anxiety and insomnia. Nightmares are a regular occurrence for me and so are sleepless nights. With the CBD/THC tinctures, I manage these well. My diagnosing doctor believed the bi-polar disorder was brought on by trauma. I now believe that if our brain can be wired to change from trauma, we can rewire it back to health through deep, intensive self-care. It took me many years for this chemical change in my brain to take place, and it's still not perfect, but it's far better than anything I ever thought possible, especially after multiple doctors told me I would be medicated for life.

Self-care for me happens in a multitude of ways, and I wanted to share what works for me. Meditation is huge. It took me years to get this into my routine regularly, but I now hardly ever skip a day. I know that one of the biggest reasons I can go without medication is because of my daily meditation routine. We now practice as a family. My husband and my eight and nine year olds join me in the living room every night at 8:30 after baby Kayden has gone down for the night. We do a guided meditation together for anywhere from ten to twenty minutes. I will also meditate on my own at times when I feel my stress and/or anxiety is getting high. I find it really helpful when working through difficult emotions.

This book started out with me in a guided meditation with my friend Natalie. We were in her home as she was hosting a women's circle I attend once per month. A few months after that first session, I went back there, and we spoke about our childhoods before going into meditation. Feelings of anger arose as we started the meditation, and Natalie asked us to sit with it and wait for it to pass. I remember thinking, *Natalie and her hokey-pokey bullshit; this is stupid.* Sitting there feeling angry, I started repeating, *angry, angry, angry.* Feeling the anger and immersing myself in it was the method; as we approached the end of the meditation, the feeling began to lift. I couldn't believe it. Sitting in it and feeling it helped me move through it! This was a real eye opener for me on how meditation works. Now, I have tried this again and not been as successful. Sometimes, we move through emotions slower than other times. Sitting in it and being mindful of how we are feeling, good or bad, is a tool. It helps us cultivate acceptance of difficult emotions. I highly recommend trying meditation in place of grabbing a drink, getting high, zoning out with TV or social media, or overeating. All of these vices are very common ways to distract ourselves or cover up feelings that we don't want to feel.

Yoga also has been a great way to help me connect to my self as well as become more mindful. I have been practicing for nineteen years—yes, even as an addict. Yoga forces you to sit with yourself for sixty to ninety minutes focusing on your physical body and on controlling your mind. Learning to be quiet when in Savasana, a resting pose, as well as while in a challenging pose, is a great life lesson. We can take this tool off of our mat and apply it to our real-world problems. Learning to focus on your breath as a tool to keep yourself calm is a way to go deeper into your physical body and your mind. There are many different types of yoga, and I highly recommend you try them all. Restorative helps you to regenerate on a cellular level, Yin helps you to open up your joints and ligaments, Vinyasa builds heat and strength in the body, and Kundalini is a deep spiritual practice. There are many more, but the ones listed here are my favourites, and I use each one for a different purpose as well as to help keep balance in my practice. If you haven't tried meditating or yoga yet, then I suggest you start with yoga, as you will get a meditative practice in it naturally.

Being active for me is a must. If I take too much time off from physical activity, I start to feel anxious; I need that release of endorphins. I also need the sense of accomplishment that comes from getting it done. Having a regular form of exercise you enjoy is a must. For me, cycling, doing functional training in the gym, and practicing yoga fulfill that. Get out and try something new if you hate what you're doing or aren't doing anything at all. Setting that routine and having the release will change your life.

Another life-changing practice I've already gone into great detail about is finding a support group that is a great fit for you. Having support in multiple areas of your life is really important. I rely on my husband for support, and I have my closest friends, my support group that is full of close friends as well, and then I also have my cycling team. Don't be afraid to be vulnerable in different areas of your life. Having multiple support systems keeps me balanced and doesn't force me to lean on only one or two people. It's really powerful.

Reading books written by women who have overcome shame is huge for me as well. I was first inspired to write this book after reading Glennon Doyle's *Love Warrior*. She is so raw and real and really lends her courage to others to show up in their lives. On days when I'm struggling with fear and shame—yes, they still live inside of me—I put on Brene Brown's Netflix special or a Ted Talk and fall into her words. She paves the way for us to find courage when all we want to do is hide. I've read most of her books and highly recommend them. She is another trailblazer for humans to rise up. I also find a lot of strength and encouragement from Gabby Bernstein's work. She has great books on meditation, spirituality, and leading with an open heart. These are three of the women I turn to when I need to step out of fear and continue on into my wholehearted life.

Setting ourselves up to be financially secure was a huge role in recovery. Lowering the amount of stress in our lives is key to good mental health, and money is a huge stressor on folks. Living within our means must be practiced. Trying to keep up with what we see on TV or social media is a recipe for disaster. I believe in envisioning exactly the way you want your life to look financially, creating vision boards, and writing it out. Believing in yourself and your financial security must be practiced daily. I like to spend time during meditation picturing myself living my life exactly as I want. Practice feeling good about money and letting go of any fearful feelings you may have around it.

Always be willing to try something new. If what you are doing isn't working, get creative and spend time cultivating new ideas. For example, I never thought about writing this book five years ago. After some time practicing creativity and meditating, I came up with the idea of writing it and creating a new possible income doing something I enjoy. All you need to do is plant the seed and have an open mind. Ideas will come to you. Play around with them, and what you come up with may completely surprise you. I believe there is abundance for all. If we can release fear and practice gratitude, there is a whole new world out there waiting for us.

Lastly, let love in. Love yourself and love others. I practice loving myself by all the things mentioned above. Eating a plant-based diet makes me feel great and gives me the maximum amount of nutrition for a healthy body and mind. Cooking is a passion, and I decided to share my favourite recipes through a cookbook. It was another opportunity for me to use something I love and create an income from it. I believe in giving back and I do that through my cycling team, which our property management company sponsors along with many other great companies. Ten percent of the profits from this book and my cookbook will go into the team, so thank you for helping me give back.

I hope that this book inspires you to live your best life, and I hope you understand that we can stumble 1,000 times and still rise up to do something great.

Love,
Dee

Acknowledgments

Thank you to my husband, Jonathan: you have been my rock through this journey, and I feel so incredibly blessed to share this life with you.

Love and blessings to my four beautiful children. You each have made me stretch and grow to be the best mother I can be. Each of you holds a mirror up for me to see myself in depths I may otherwise not recognize. I love you all dearly and deeply for eternity.

Thank you to my wonderful therapist, Cindy. You helped me see something in myself I didn't believe existed. Your vulnerability allowed me to try one more time to open my heart and share my gifts with the world.

My Soul Sisters, Amy, Brandy, Emilie, Hayley, Holly, Kerry, Kim, Stephanie, and Thea—thank you for lending me your strength and insight. Seeing myself through your eyes has allowed me to Rise Up. Shakti Sisters for life.

Dear Natalie, you are magic. Your light shines bright upon everyone you meet. Thank you for joining me on this journey. Full Circle ... hOMe.

A heartfelt thanks to my best friend, Thyra. You've been by my side for almost two decades. Our friendship gives me comfort and feels like home.

Thank you to my parents and siblings. We offer each other lessons on forgiveness and acceptance. I believe this divine work has been a master class on personal growth.

A shout-out to my teammates: thank you for believing in me and sticking through when times were dark. Paolina, you inspire and motivate me to be better constantly and consistently.

Jordana, thank you for your friendship, guidance, and support. You give me clarity and hope.

Thank you, Katie and Tina, for your beautiful editing and for helping me move this book along. Nickole, you have a creative gift. Thank you for guiding me and helping me create beautiful work.

Cheers to everyone who has shared a vulnerable story with me along the way. Unknowingly, you have offered me courage to amplify my own voice.

Thank you everyone who I have crossed paths with. The good and the bad experiences have all shaped who I am and what I have to offer in this beautiful world.

About the Author

Deirdre Maloney is the founder of High Gate Racing, Canada's largest all female competitive cycling team. She raises money for their youth development program and advocates for women in sport. Also the co-founder of a women's support group in her own community, Deirdre believes in sharing our stories to cultivate more collective healing. Deirdre lives in Ontario, Canada, with her husband and children. Read more of her work at theunfoldingproject.com

Read more from Deirdre at

The Unfolding Project

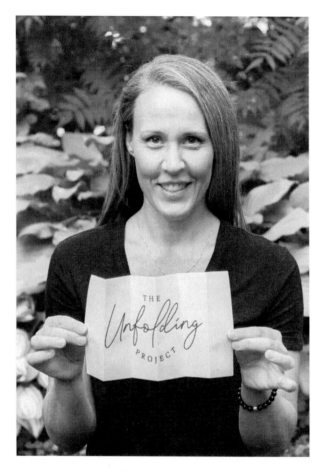

theunfoldingproject.com

Facebook: @deirdremaloney01
Instagram: @deirdremaloney_

Thank you

for supporting HighGate Racing.
Ten percent of the profits from this book goes to our team.

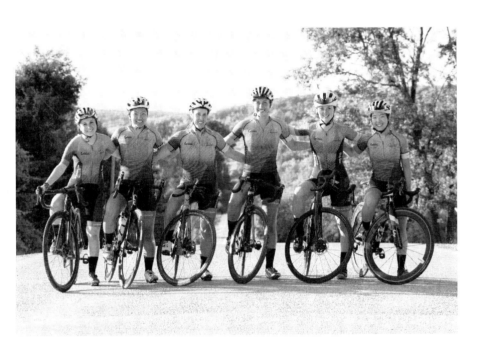

For more information about
the team go to highgatecycling.com

Facebook: @highgateracing
Instagram: @highgateracing

Coming Soon...

Healthy Mind Healthy Body
Plant Based Cookbook for the family

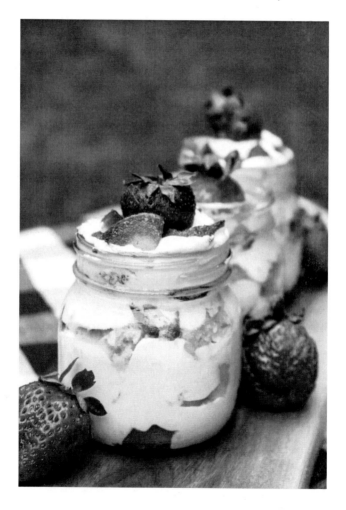

Find out more at deemaloney.com